The Natural Supplement & Nutrition Guide

For every stage of life

First published in Great Britain in 2025
by Laurence King, an imprint of
The Orion Publishing Group Ltd, Carmelite House,
50 Victoria Embankment, London EC4Y 0DZ

An Hachette UK Company

10 9 8 7 6 5 4 3 2 1

A CIP catalogue record for this book is available
from the British Library.

ISBN (Hardback) 978 1 39960 301 0
ISBN (eBook) 978 1 39960 302 7

Origination by F1 Colour
Printed in China by C&C Offset Printing Co. Ltd

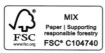

www.laurenceking.com
www.orionbooks.co.uk

The Natural Supplement & Nutrition Guide

For every stage of life

Henrietta
Norton

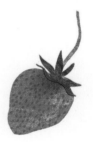

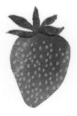

LAURENCE KING

Contents

Introduction 6
How to Use this Book 10

PART ONE: UNDERSTANDING NUTRITION *12*
Why aren't we getting the right nutrients? *14*
Why do we take supplements? *20*
Why do supplements need to be natural? *21*
How to choose supplements *27*
How to build the foundations of a healthy diet *29*
Preparing food *39*

PART TWO: MAXIMISING HEALTH AT EVERY AGE *44*
Introduction *46*
Birth to Early Puberty *47*
– Infancy: 0–12 months *47*
– Toddler and preschool: 1–4 years *49*
– School children: 5–12 years *51*
Adolescence: 12–19 years *57*
Young Adulthood to Middle Years *69*
Middle Years to Wiser Years *76*

**PART THREE:
SUPPLEMENTS FOR COMMON COMPLAINTS** *90*
Introduction *92*
Skin Health *95*
– Acne *96*
– Eczema *96*
– Psoriasis *97*
– Lifestyle and diet to support skin health *98*

A Healthy Mind *101*
- Stress and anxiety *102*
- Low mood and depression *104*
- Tiredness and fatigue *105*
- Difficulty sleeping *106*
- Memory *111*
- Lifestyle and diet to support mood, energy and sleep *112*

Body Health *121*
- Digestion *122*
- Osteoporosis and osteopenia *128*
- Joint pain *132*
- Cholesterol support *139*

General Health *146*
- Cold and flu *146*
- Hay fever *151*

Women's Health *159*
- Endometriosis and adenomyosis *160*
- Menstrual imbalances *166*
- PCOS *170*
- Perimenopause and menopause *175*

Fertility *184*

Pregnancy and Early Motherhood *192*

References 202
Further Reading 204
Index 205
Acknowledgements 208

Introduction

All living things rely on receiving the right nutrients from their environment to allow them to survive and flourish. Humans are no different. Our incredible bodies evolved over millennia to consume and absorb foods that are found in nature, and despite our species' incredible ability to progress and innovate, we will always need nature to provide the nutrients our bodies require for life and good health.

Often, these days, we hear science and nature spoken or written about as different things. The 'natural approach' is placed in opposition to 'the scientific approach' as if they are opposing forces. But I believe that a natural approach and a scientific approach are often one and the same thing. Nature has been our greatest scientist from the beginning of time; what we call science is simply the study of that which is all around us, with the aim of understanding nature's processes and optimising them for our use.

Ideally, we would get all of the nutrients we need for strong bodies and minds through a healthy, balanced diet – just as humans have been doing since the beginning of history, as we evolved in nature. But for many reasons, which I will go on to discuss, this is challenging in our modern world.

Eating wholesome, high-quality and nutrient-rich food is the primary way to support good health. We are empowered to make daily choices that impact our wellbeing and, if we are also shopping or cooking for others, those around us too. But more than this, the benefit of a wholesome diet goes beyond the nutrients it provides by offering a means to commune, share, celebrate, connect with others – a higher purpose for food that is valued in traditional cultures and one we need to be reminded of in a modern, often less connected lifestyle, in which food has become more functional than soulful, more reductive than whole.

But on the plus side, many of us are increasingly seeing our health as something to be actively supported and maintained, rather than taken for granted until it becomes a problem. In the last decade, there has been a resurgence of interest in nutritional therapy, as more people have started to understand that health niggles are so often the body telling us it does not have some essential vitamin or mineral that it needs.

For over two decades, I have worked with food supplements, within the industry as a formulator and also as a nutritional practitioner. During this time, I have seen the tremendous results that can come from supplements when they are used as part of a programme for wellbeing. These days, I find that I am asked similar questions about natural nutrition more and more often:

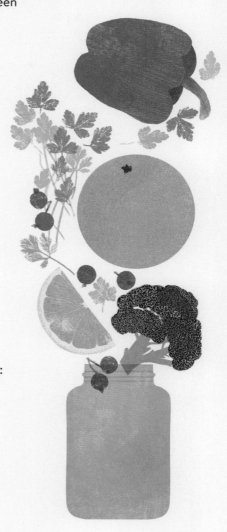

* Why do I need to take supplements?

* How can I sleep better?

* What is the best way of dealing with fatigue and lack of energy?

* How can I improve my digestion?

* How should I be supporting my immune system?

* How can a ensure I am getting the right nutrients to support my life stage?

* What are the benefits of natural supplements?

The reality is that while many of us are taking a more proactive approach to our own health, the information available can be confusing or contradictory, and the conversation often feels dominated by big companies with products to sell. I have seen first-hand how many people are looking for sound information in a myth-saturated and often overwhelming sea. If you have picked up this book it is likely that you also feel the same. You may be starting from zero knowledge or you may have a good understanding of nutrition or supplements but still feel confused. In this book, I will offer advice and information that will help you to feel clearer on some of these questions. It aims to provide solution-based approaches to health, offering accessible, practical and curated advice for everyday wellbeing.

I first became interested in nutrition specifically in my mid-twenties because of my own health issues, though in many ways I have always felt drawn to holistic wellbeing and particularly our relationship with food and nature. I worked as a formulator within the supplement industry for a number of years, which gave me an insight into what goes into commercially made supplements and how synthetic nutrients are created. This was illuminating, as it was so far removed from how we know nutrients work in food and, importantly, how bodies have been designed to receive and process them. These things just didn't seem to add up and I felt strongly that we needed to find a way of retaining the natural nutrients found in food in supplement form. I found it uncomfortable that the synthetic nutrient market was misleading customers into thinking their products were natural but, more than this, I knew that natural nutrients had health advantages over synthetic forms, which we were missing out on. I became committed, both as a nutritional practitioner and a regular supplement taker, to using only the most naturally sourced nutrients. It is also where my company Wild Nutrition began, with the aim of creating natural nutrients and products backed by science, which would bring the benefits that synthetic supplements simply weren't able to provide, as well as respecting our innate relationship with food for deep nourishment and health. My background in working as a nutritional therapist also allowed me to see how 'real' people need and use supplements, what works and what doesn't. This is important, as many supplements are created by scientists behind desks or in labs without a connection to real needs.

It is not an exaggeration to say that natural nutrition, along with natural supplementation, has been life-changing for my family and me. On a day-to-day basis in supporting energy, tolerance of stress, digestion and defences against seasonal bugs, but also through life stages such as early childhood and teenage ages for our children and fertility, pregnancy and now menopause for me. It has also been powerful enough to turn around my diagnosis of endometriosis where I was given a prognosis of being on prescription drugs long term, with a very slim chance of being able to conceive. By harnessing the power of nutrition and supplementation, I went on to have three healthy pregnancies and children.

Even the very best quality natural supplements can never be a magic cure for all that ails us, and nor can they replace our foundational relationship with wholesome food. What I hope to show you in the course of this book is how both our diet and supplementation work in synergy to build good health. I also feel strongly that no guru or health expert can replace your own relationship with your body. Sometimes we may need support with the knowledge of what is happening in our bodies and an understanding of how to respond to their needs, but it is always down to us to listen, engage with and take ownership of our health. The more we engage with our nutrition and become consciously aware of the needs of our bodies and how we are supplying these needs, the better, and my hope is that this book will support this process.

Health is holistic and so we will also explore the important influence that sleep and rest, stress, exercise and emotional and spiritual balance have on our overall health too.

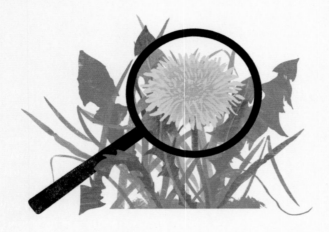

How to use the book

This book is designed both as an introduction to the principles of natural nutrition and a guide that can be kept on the bookshelf and used as a point of reference throughout the years. The information is here to inform and empower you – and should be enough to give you the confidence to embark on or continue your journey into nutrition-focused wellbeing. It is not a scientific guide to nutrition nor indeed supplements, but it may be the foundation on which you build an interest to know more. If you do feel you would like to go deeper, I have made some recommendations for further reading on various topics at the end of the book.

PART ONE:

However you wish to use this book and whatever has brought you here, I recommend that you start by reading Part One from start to finish. This section of the book explains the foundational principles of developing a conscious relationship with nutrition as well as outlining some simple, sustainable methods you can adopt to create change straight away. Here you will find an in-depth look at what supplements are, why and when we should take them, and why natural is key. There is also information on how to cook vegetables to best preserve their nutrients, seasonality, and what we mean when we say 'eating with a nourishing mindset'.

PART TWO:

Here we will look at the different life stages – birth to puberty, teens to twenties, young adulthood to middle years and middle years to the wiser years – and the changing nutritional needs we experience within each phase. I will explain the key factors to be aware of to help you to eat and supplement your diet to best support your needs at that time.

PART THREE:

This section has been written as a handy reference guide for you to dip into as and when you need. It seeks to offer natural solutions for specific health niggles or concerns at any age, ranging from acne and digestive issues to hormonal or memory concerns.

Above all, I hope that the principles and information within this book offer you encouragement and empowerment to use food and natural approaches for good health throughout your life, and that our relationship with food and natural world will help and inspire you to look after yourself in body, mind and soul.

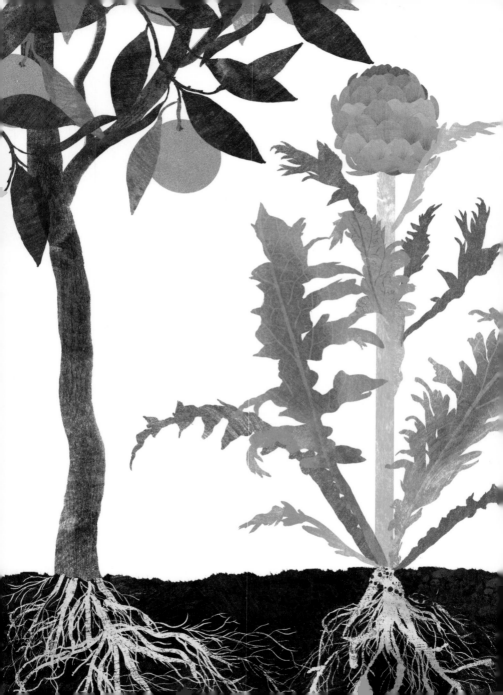

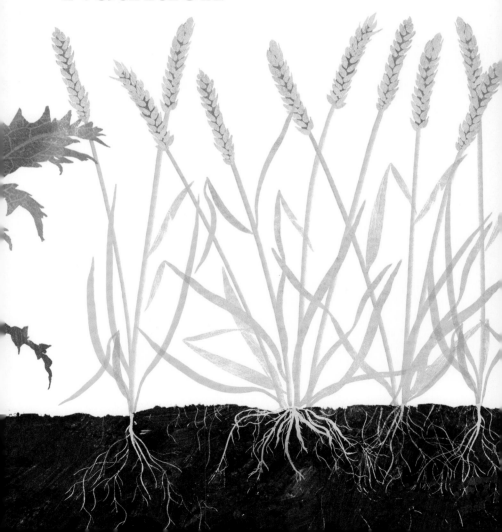

PART ONE
Understanding Nutrition

Why aren't we getting the right nutrients?

I often hear it said that we don't need to take supplements if we are eating a balanced diet. But while it is true that wholesome food is the foundation on which we build our health, food supplements can have a fundamental part to play in living well, protecting against stress, and bridging the gap between feeling OK and feeling well. In our modern world, there are several factors that are muddying a once simple and still crucial relationship with good food.

WHAT ARE VITAMINS AND MINERALS?

Vitamins and minerals belong to a group of nutrients called micronutrients, so called because they are needed in comparatively small amounts compared to another group called macronutrients, which include protein, fat and carbohydrates. Although vitamins and minerals are nutrients your body needs in small amounts, they are essential if you are to stay healthy. In the early twentieth century, the Polish biochemist Casimir Funk discovered the first set of 'micronutrient structures' within food. He termed these compounds vitamins (*vita* for life and *amines* as the term used to describe organic compounds that are organised around nitrogen). These special molecules were isolated from foods and became the new heroes of health, providing cures for diseases known to be caused by nutritional deficiencies, such as scurvy or beriberi.

Within food, vitamins are created by the plant itself, whereas minerals are drawn into the plant from the soil and water. When found in their natural environments, vitamins and minerals are made up of interconnected parts, like those in a jigsaw puzzle, that work as a 'team' to nourish and protect the plant (and therefore us when we consume them). All pieces are needed to achieve the full benefit of a particular vitamin or mineral.

1. Our food doesn't contain the nutrients it once did

Findings show that we can no longer rely on our food to supply us with the full range and quantity of the vital nutrients we require for optimum health. Over a decade ago, a report from the Department of Environment, Food and Rural Affairs (DEFRA) stated that the trace minerals in UK fruit and vegetables had fallen by over 76 per cent over the last 50 years.

Even as long ago as 1936, the US Senate recognised the growing depletion of nutrients in our soils worldwide and published a report stating that: 'The alarming fact is that foods (fruit, vegetables and grains) are now being raised on millions of acres of land that no longer contain enough of certain minerals and are therefore starving us – no matter how much of them we eat. No man of today can eat enough fruit and vegetables to supply his system with the minerals he requires for perfect health.'

We know that many of the foods we eat have been grown on exhausted, nutrient-depleted soil, caused by a monoculture system, use of chemical sprays and poor crop rotation. Industrial farming practices have narrowed the biodiversity of the land our food grows or grazes on, and therefore the health of the soil, and then, ultimately, us. If the key minerals that are used by plants as building blocks to make the vitamins and minerals that we require are not present in the soil, then they will not be found in the food we eat.

In addition to this, we know that – especially in the UK but in many other places too – we eat a lot of imported 'fresh' foods. In reality, they are picked before they are ripe and transported in refrigerated containers for many miles to reach us. We have all experienced the difference in taste between a fruit or vegetable picked ripe from the source and those from packets – and it's not just the taste that is affected. It may look good on the supermarket shelves but this produce lacks much-needed vitamins and minerals, along with flavour. This way of producing food is causing a strain on our human health as well as the planet's. So even a 'healthy' or organic diet can fall short of providing the full nutrition we need. This is often a large part of the reason why even those of us who try our best to proactively eat well are still suffering health niggles and issues that we can't seem to shake.

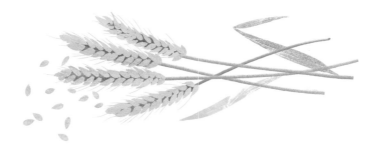

2. We follow a Western diet

In the West, our diet can be generally characterised by a high proportion of energy-dense foods. We have easy access to ultra-processed food, often with high amounts of sugars, salt and trans fats. This is made worse by a limited amount and diversity of vegetables, fruits, wholegrains and therefore fibre and nutrients. There's strong scientific evidence that shows a causative relationship between these foods and the development of chronic diseases, including diabetes, cancer and depression (Srour et al., 2021).

In the West, we have a population with increased access to food but one that is, on the whole, both overfed and malnourished.

The National Diet and Nutrition Survey carried out by Public Health England and the Food Standards Agency in 2019 found that:

* 19 per cent of children and 13 per cent of adults were deficient in vitamin D

* 17 per cent of children and 19 per cent of women of childbearing age were deficient in folate, a key nutrient for healthy foetal development, the normal function of the immune system and psychological wellbeing

* 8 out of 10 adults were deficient in omega 3 – linked to many health conditions, including depression, learning difficulties and cardiovascular problems

* the average intake of saturated fat was 13.1 per cent per capita, compared to the recommended less than 10 per cent

* the average intake of free sugars was 9.4 per cent of daily energy intake, versus the recommendation of less than 5 per cent

What is galling is that many of us will be consuming these health-sapping foods unknowingly. Food processing techniques have progressed at a rapid rate in the last century, placing the onus on convenience, low cost (to the manufacturer, at least) and palatability. Lack of taste and substance is masked by highly refined sugars and flavourings, while the use of synthetically generated stabilisers increases shelf life. This industrial approach to food production has had a big impact on our relationship with food, which is now a profit-making commodity for the manufacturers. It has changed our expectations of what food should taste and look like, and has altered our taste buds to expect foods higher in sugar and salt to initiate enjoyment.

3. Our diets are not sufficiently diverse

As in plant life, diversity is key when it comes to a wholesome diet. Even when we make an effort to eat healthily, we may be consuming a narrower range of nutrients than we realise. The nature of our busy lives means that we often fall back on the same dinners week in, week out, eat leftovers for multiple meals and stick to our favourite snacks. We can be ticking off five-plus portions of veg a day, but these are often the same ones, meaning our diets can end up excessively heavy in some vitamins and minerals but deficient in others.

4. Our nutrient needs are changing

As we get older, our need for vitamins and minerals will change, as will the amount of nutrients our body can synthesise itself or absorb. In addition, life stages such as pregnancy, menopause or illness can increase or change our need for certain nutrients, as can exposure to stress and environmental pollutants. The growth of research into nutrigenomics (how our genetics responds to nutrition) has shown a need for greater consideration for the distinct nutritional needs of different stages of life and different genders.

5. Prescription medicines are on the rise

The UK government initiated an independent review of national overprescribing in 2021, which found that 15 per cent of the population is taking five or more medicines a day. We know that pharmaceutical medication, including the contraceptive pill, anti-inflammatory medication and antacids, can impact how we absorb or break down nutrients needed for good health, but they can also increase the body's need for important nutrients. An example of this is protein pump inhibitor (PPI) medication, taken for acid reflux, often by those who have stomach ulcers. PPI medication can increase the risk of vitamin B12 deficiency, a member of the B vitamin family needed for cognitive function and energy.

As a nation, we are taking a lot of medication, and yet the study found that 10 per cent of the volume of prescription items dispensed through primary care in England is either inappropriate for that patient's circumstances and wishes, or the patient's needs could be better served with alternative treatments. One in five hospital admissions over the age of 65 are caused by the adverse effects of medicines. In all, 1.1 billion prescriptions were dispensed last year – a rise of 47 per cent in a decade.

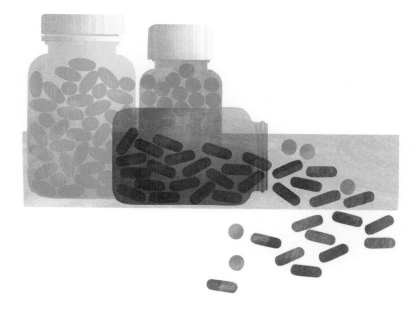

Why do we take supplements?

All of these factors taken together means that there is so often a gap between the nutrients we require and what we are getting through our food. Supplements can help to bridge this increasing gap, even when eating a healthy diet. This is especially true during times of illness, regular intense exercise and during pregnancy and breastfeeding, as examples. If you follow a vegetarian or vegan diet, you may also find it harder to access all required nutrients, especially iron and vitamin B12. In these cases, supplements are also recommended.

I have found that many of us have had marginally sufficient levels of nutrients in order to 'tick over' throughout our lives so far. However, there is a vast difference between ticking over and feeling your best. It can be easy to accept regular colds, bloating or hormonal imbalances as just something that happens to you, but really, if your body is working well, these experiences should and could be few and far between.

So, for many of us, supplements can play a functional role in our everyday wellbeing, helping us to feel well in our daily lives, along with preventing or reducing our chances of developing longer term, more chronic conditions. However, not all supplements are the same, and with so many on the market, it can be hard to know which are right for you. To complicate matters further, nutrients are manufactured differently. Broadly, these different approaches fall into two categories: the natural way or the highly processed way. Just as with ultra-processed (synthetic) foods and more natural whole foods, the benefits of these two processes can be very different. It is my hope, therefore, that the information provided in this chapter will empower you to make the right choice for you and your body.

Why do supplements need to be natural?

While the discoveries of scientists such as Casimir Funk offered pioneering treatment of some nasty conditions, the unintended consequence was that it marked a shift in our relationship with food. As popularity for supplementation rose, in part due to food shortages caused by the Second World War, there was increased demand to make vitamin supplements cheaper and production more scalable. By the mid-twentieth century, these natural compounds were no longer being extracted from food, but synthetically created within a laboratory. The problem with this highly processed or synthetic method is that it misses many of the components found in a 'natural' nutrient. As a result, the nutrients it creates bear little resemblance to the structure of a nutrient as we would find it in food. It also strips out many of the other components, or pieces of the jigsaw puzzle, that help us absorb the nutritional benefits. This is why prominent researchers have continually championed for nutrients to be found in their natural form in order to be most effective. Dr Albert Szent-Györgyi, who was awarded the Nobel prize for the extraction of vitamin C from paprika, stated, 'When I had crystalline ascorbic acid, we tried it on patients with scurvy, expecting a strong action. It did nothing.' In other words, despite scurvy being the result of vitamin C deficiency, and ascorbic acid being chemically the same as vitamin C, the isolated nutrient did not provide the same result, regardless of increasing the dose.

The best way for humans to obtain vitamin C, therefore, is through diet, and plant foods represent the best primary source.

What are highly processed or synthetic nutrients?

Both vitamins and minerals can be manufactured synthetically to recreate the chemical structure of any given vitamin or mineral found in food. Indeed, this is the most common production method, thanks to its low cost and scalability. Production is dominated by three large pharmaceutical companies – La Roche, AEC and BASF – all of whom can produce on a vast scale.

As we have seen, a good example of the synthetic approach is vitamin C. The structure of vitamin C in its natural state includes over 20 different compounds, the majority of which are a group of plant chemicals called ascorbates. One of these, known as ascorbic acid, has been identified as one of the most 'active' parts of the vitamin C jigsaw. For this reason, manufacturers of these highly processed nutrients focus on reproducing ascorbic acid alone, by mixing corn starch with sorbitol, and frequently label it, misleadingly, as vitamin C.

But what of the other components in the jigsaw puzzle? Where are they at the end of this highly processed method? There are many who believe that there is no difference between the natural nutrient and the synthetic version, that the body does not know the difference. However, an increasing number of professionals and consumers, encouraged by research, are challenging this approach and seeking a more natural production method.

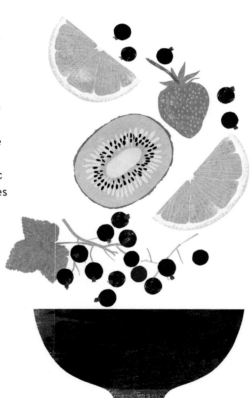

BIOAVAILABILITY

Bioavailability and absorption are often used to describe the same thing, but there is a slight difference between the two. Bioavailability refers to the amount and speed at which a substance is broken down (or metabolised), absorbed and then transported to the cells in the body that require it, where it is therefore available to initiate a cellular change. Absorption refers only to the stage where a substance is metabolised and absorbed, and not to the all-important transportation stage.

What this means in practice is that a nutrient may be shown in scientific studies to be well 'absorbed' but this doesn't necessarily mean that it has good 'bioavailability' (i.e. is effectively transported to the cells that require it). The best way to tell whether most nutrients are both better absorbed *and* bioavailable is to measure the amount of a nutrient in the bloodstream over time – preferably 72 hours or more. A longer period of time is preferable because it can separate those forms that might be absorbed quickly but do not sustain their effect, from those that absorb more steadily and sustainably (the latter being preferable to initiate cellular change and, ultimately, benefit our health).

Sometimes the two terms can be misused within the supplement industry, with claims that their product is more 'bioavailable' when the data is actually only looking at the rate of absorption. This is another consideration that should inform your choices.

What are natural nutrients?

In contrast to highly processed synthetic nutrients, natural nutrients reflect the more comprehensive structure of a nutrient as it is found in nature – i.e., the full jigsaw – and therefore offer an advantage over synthetic forms. Not only in terms of the health benefits but also as a way of respecting the innate relationship that our bodies have with natural food and its connection to our wellbeing, which can never be superseded, despite our scientific advances.

A good example of the co-dependent relationship between our health and nature is seen by looking at how plants process nutrients on our behalf. The root system of a plant draws minerals from the soil – calcium carbonate, for example – into the plant's cells. These minerals are then metabolised by the plant, converting them into plant-bound forms that we can then process easily once we eat them. Crucially, this clever natural process within plant life removes unwanted material (like the carbonate in calcium carbonate, for example) that we would not be able to process effectively.

Humans and (most) animals can't, obviously, eat soil and transform nutrients within it into a form that our bodies can use – hence the historic need to obtain our vitamins and minerals through food. This is a very basic but powerful and awe-inspiring example of our reliance on nature.

Natural nutrients – as opposed to highly processed, synthetic recreations of chemicals found in plants – are created by replicating this plant process within a controlled laboratory setting. This generates nutrients in a form that our bodies can recognise and use with ease. Not only is this approach intuitive and respectful to our relationship with nature, but it has also been shown in scientific literature to have health advantages too. Perhaps you can understand why I am so committed to this way and why we use only natural nutrients at Wild Nutrition.

When I started my business, over 99 per cent of the supplement market comprised highly processed products and I was tentative (but not put off!) about how our approach would be received by both consumers and the industry. Our vision, which we labelled our Food-Grown® philosophy, was born of the belief that the best form of nutrition is the food nature provides. Essentially, the Food-Grown® philosophy is ultimately one of reverence for our innate connection to nature. To our surprise, the message we wanted to deliver about the value of natural nutrients seemed to make immediate intuitive sense to many, and increasingly so. I suppose it's not that much more challenging to understand than the fact that ultra-processed foods and ready meals have a different health value to wholefoods.

Our Food-Grown® philosophy and process

At the root of the Food-Grown® philosophy is a commitment to capturing nutrients in their 'whole' form, using a manufacturing technology that replicates the natural process within plants. The process was pioneered by Andrew Szalay, a pharmacist and researcher at the same institution as Dr Szent-Györgyi, to optimise the absorption of vitamins and minerals through food but without the bulk of wholefood.

In this process, all vitamins and minerals are 'fed' into appropriate live food cells, such as citrus, carrot, cabbage, alfalfa, baker's yeast or probiotics. Which cell to use is decided by what is most naturally suited to the nutrient or mineral – so citrus pulp for vitamin C, carrot concentrate for beta-carotene and so on. As in nature, this food cell then metabolises and re-natures the vitamin or mineral into a more natural but complex structure that the body recognises and uses more effectively. This sophisticated, targeted delivery means that lower dosing can be therapeutic.

Food-Grown® nutrients have also been shown to produce benefits that are not available with synthetic isolated forms. Vitamin B12 in a Food-Grown® form, for example, has been shown to overcome pernicious anaemia in conditions where the synthetic form of vitamin B12 is ineffective (Vinson & Bose, 1988).

MORE DOES NOT EQUAL MORE
(OR THE HORMESIS EFFECT)

It is commonly assumed that if a little of something is good for us, then surely more is even better. This is not true for many things, such as stress or alcohol! Supplements are no different, especially synthetic supplements. Our body is continually working to create homeostasis – that delicate balance between things to regulate key functions, such as blood glucose levels or body temperature. Its regulation of vitamins and minerals is no different and if one is too high, the body will work to correct this (usually by excreting the excess of the nutrient through our urine). For example, a single dose of synthetic ascorbic acid or vitamin C higher than 200mg will reduce the absorption of the nutrient to 50 per cent and cause the excess to be excreted. Which is work for the body and a waste of money for us too. Toxicity, especially of fat-soluble nutrients (such as vitamins A, D, E and K) consumed in high doses, is also a concern, as is 'competitive absorption' whereby high doses of calcium can inhibit the absorption of other minerals such as zinc, magnesium and iron in some cases. Having chronically high levels of one nutrient can create imbalances elsewhere in the body (Goggins & Matten, 2012).

It is actually a very smart and beneficial safety mechanism of the body – which, as we know, is a complex and sophisticated machine that thrives off balance. What we want to do, therefore, when we choose supplementation is to support the body in its natural quest to attain and maintain balance, not flood it with a particular nutrient. I believe this to be not only an efficacious approach to nutritional health, but a way of respecting the natural sophistication of the inner workings of all our bodies.

How to choose supplements

One of the main factors that deters people from trying supplements to help with health concerns is the large number of products available. Reading labels can be a minefield and even those with good intent can be confused by natural or 'clean' looking packaging or vague statements. If you have spent time in health food stores, supermarkets or online, you will have noticed that it seems there is a supplement for almost anything. And this choice can be overwhelming. Not only are they available in a multitude of forms, such as capsules, tablets, powders, gummies, liquid or patches, but there is an array of different prices and manufacturing processes used. Supplements also stretch way beyond the simple line-up of vitamins and minerals now too and can include essential fatty acids such as omega 3 or omega 6, herbs, medicinal mushrooms, 'superfoods' or amino acids.

Understanding the measurements

In the UK, the Department of Health established the concept of recommended daily allowances (RDA) in 1979. This was done as a response to increasing evidence that nutrient deficiencies in our diets were causing health problems. Guidelines were therefore set for 13 vitamins and 14 minerals, based on EU guidance levels on the average daily amount that the 'average healthy person' needs to consume per day to prevent a deficiency. Recently, RDAs have been replaced by nutrient reference values (NRV). This may be why you have seen references to both RDAs and/or NRVs on labels, but they are, essentially, the same thing.

Food supplement labels list the ingredients included in the product and give the proportion of the NRV value (as a percentage of the total NRV recommended per day) that is contained within the supplement. So for example, the NRV of vitamin C is 80mg, so a product that provides 40mg of vitamin C per recommended dose would be listed as 50 per cent of the NRV. Nutrients are measured in grams, micrograms, milligrams or international units.

Although standardising the requirement and value of a nutrient helps to improve regulation and guidelines, it is far from perfect. Who is the average person, for one? (There will be differences between the needs of a 16-year-old and a 60-year-old, for example.) And are we looking merely to prevent deficiency or are we seeking wellbeing and preventative approaches to create long-term health? So although this serves as a baseline, they need to be considered more individually, taking into account age, current health, diet and lifestyle factors such as how much stress we are under or the quantity and/or type of exercise we do. This is more reflective of the holistic nature of our wellbeing and of nutrition too, where supplements and a nourishing balanced diet can form the foundation of a multifactorial picture.

NUTRITIONAL INFORMATION	2 capsules provide:	% NRV*
Vitamin D (as D3)	1.5µg	30
Vitamin E	5mg α-TE	42
Vitamin K	10µg	13
Vitamin C	30mg	38
Thiamin (Vitamin B1)	1.4mg	127
Riboflavin (Vitamin B2)	1.6mg	114
Niacin	5mg NE	31
Vitamin B6	5mg	357
Folic Acid	60µg	30
Vitamin B12	1µg	40
Biotin	45µg	90
Pantothenic Acid	5mg	83
Calcium	60mg	8
Magnesium	30mg	8
Iron	3mg	21
Zinc	5mg	50
Copper	0.5mg	50
Manganese	1mg	50
Selenium	100µg	182
Chromium (from Chromium GTF)	50µg	125
Molybdenum	10µg	20
Iodine	20µg	13
Choline	2.5mg	
Inositol	10mg	
Alpha Lipoic Acid	10mg	
Beta-Carotene	1.5mg	
Bioflavonoids	3mg	
Beetroot powder	50mg	
Ashwagandha powder	200mg	

*NRV - Nutrient Reference Value
µg - Microgram, mg - Miligram, α-TE - Alpha-tocopherol equivalents, NE - Niacin Equivalents, GTF - Glucose Tolerance Factor

FOOD SUPPLEMENT WITH VITAMINS MINERALS AND ASHWAGANDHA

CHECK FOR ADDED INGREDIENTS

Check the ingredients on the labels for added fillers and binders (also called excipients). These are added to products to 'bulk' them out or bind them into tablets or capsules. These include ingredients such as anti-caking agents like magnesium stearate, silicon dioxide, potato maltodextrin, sucrose, acacia gum, microcrystalline cellulose, corn starch, and even talc. Supplement companies must list their ingredients in order of quantity on the label. Therefore, if you see these ingredients at the top of the ingredients list, you know it is more 'bulk' than substance.

How to build the foundations of a healthy diet

Sometimes change can be daunting, and especially changes that revolve around health and exercise. They can often be the preserve of New Year's resolutions or grand overhauls that we don't and can't stick to. But looking after ourselves every day can be as simple as making small, sustainable changes to the way that we cook and the foods that we choose. Keep it simple. Do small things consistently and build on this. First, work out what is right for you and your lifestyle, then decide what you can commit to now, and what you would like to be able to commit to in the near future, and work towards that. There is no need to feel overwhelmed; go gently with incremental changes that you can build on and remember, eating well is not punitive, it is an act of self-care.

Despite the great advances and research in nutritional medicine in the 20 years I have been working as a nutritional therapist, I have come to see that many of the findings still come back to traditional, naturopathic principles which have been practised for millennia. A naturopathic approach to wellbeing is one that recognises the interconnection and interdependence of all living things, viewing the body as an integrated whole. Above all, it honours the body's innate wisdom to heal and thrive. This is the ethos that I have come to see as the most intuitive way to live and also the most beneficial for the many clients I have worked with over the years, as well as my own health and that of my family.

Taking from these years of experience, the following offers some basic foundations for wellbeing that can benefit us all, no matter our life stage. Taking time for the eating experience can help us to reduce cravings, control our portion sizes and enhance our interconnectedness with the flow of people, animals and nature that contributed to the food on our plate. These foundations can enhance your mealtime to make it a deeper, more nourishing experience.

In Parts Two and Three, you will find more specific advice relevant to your health concerns and stage in life. Consider these the starting point – the building blocks upon which you can build a tailored approach to nutrition and supplementation that works for you.

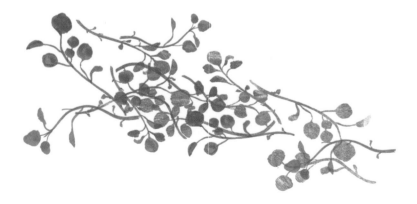

1. Eat with a nourishing mindset

Eating in a way that nourishes you does not need to be obsessive. In fact, quite the opposite. Healthy eating is an emotional and physical experience, involving all the senses. Taking the time to enjoy your food and relax around mealtimes can affect how well food is used by your body. For many, the sense of 'balance' when choosing food has been lost. Instead, food choices may be governed by counting calories or adverts suggesting that you will feel or look better if you eat a branded food. Listening to your body has taken a back seat and many women in particular feel guilt or shame around food. The reality is that our appetite changes from day to day, often for good reason. It is so important for you to listen to your body's needs and provide it with the most nutrient-dense, nourishing fuel for growth. Think quality over quantity and find pleasure in experimenting with foods you may not have chosen before.

Eat slowly, savouring your food, and give it the full attention it deserves. Chewing your food is the second significant part of digestion (thinking of and smelling food is the first step!). As much as 30–40 per cent of our digestive response to food comes from having 'awareness' when we eat. This simply means that if we do not concentrate on our food or eat mindfully, our ability to digest the food is significantly reduced. Many of us eat on the run, but it is important to avoid this as much as you can; try to make your time with food a moment of proper connection and savour it as often as you can.

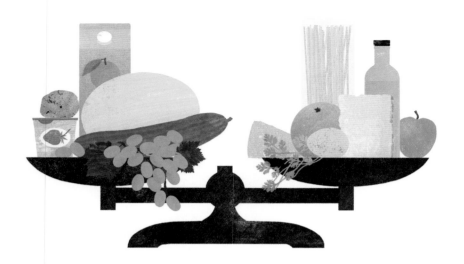

ARE YOU 'EATING' YOUR EMOTIONS?

Eat in a setting where you feel relaxed. If you are eating in the car, in front of a computer while doing work or browsing the internet, or while using your phone, your body is in 'doing' rather than 'digesting' mode and not able to give full attention to eating. As a result, you may tend to eat more or eat foods that are not healing. If you feel like you are eating to quash an 'emotion' – a phenomenon described as 'lonely mouth' in Japan – see if you can first acknowledge and express your emotions in another way. These practices will all help with the digestive process – helping you to get the most out of food.

2. Eat according to the seasons

This may seem like a far stretch given our global food sources and supermarket choices, but choosing fruit and vegetables that are in season can go a long way to helping us get the nutrients we need at the right time and, if they are locally or nationally sourced too, supporting our local economy and reducing our carbon footprint.

It is also a gradual way of connecting to the natural 'cycle of life' that is all around us – in nature but also in our food. Foods that are grown in season tend to be picked when they are ripe, which increases the nutrient value. It also means that we are more likely to be supplied with the right balance of nutrients when we need them: Mother Nature cleverly provides vegetables rich in carotenes, or berries dense in vitamin C, for immune support in the autumn, for example.

Making soups and veg-based smoothies are excellent ways of packing in the nutrients. I firmly believe that we should eat foods that are warm in the colder months and foods that are cooler in the warmer months. According to naturopathic and traditional Chinese medicine principles, eating in this way also supports digestion. During the autumn and winter season, revive the slow cooker. Low temperatures preserve many of the essential nutrients found in meat and can also make it more digestible, without destroying the benefits of the amino acids. Aside from this, the slow cooker is a practical, cost-efficient way of having a meal ready at the end of the day.

3. Eat a rainbow a day

Each day, try to sample all the colours of food, including red, orange, yellow, green and purple, to ensure that you get enough of the important phytochemicals and their health benefits. Aim for a minimum of five portions of vegetables per day and three portions of fruit of varying colours (a portion is about a handful or 80g of cooked greens, a medium-sized tomato or apple). These are just some examples of the different coloured foods you can build into your day:

Red: Red apples, beetroot, red cabbage, cherries, cranberries, pink grapefruit, red grapes, red peppers, pomegranates, red potatoes, radishes, raspberries, rhubarb, strawberries, tomatoes, watermelon

Orange: Apricots, squashes, sweet potatoes, carrots, nectarines, oranges, papayas, mangoes, peaches, persimmons, pumpkins, tangerines

Yellow-green: Green apples, artichokes, asparagus, avocados, green beans, broccoli, Brussels sprouts, green cabbage, cucumbers, rainbow chard, green grapes, kiwi, lettuce, lemons, limes, green onions, peas, green pepper, spinach, courgette

Blue-purple: Purple kale and purple sprouting broccoli, purple cabbage, purple potatoes, aubergine, purple grapes, blueberries, blackberries, boysenberries, figs, plums

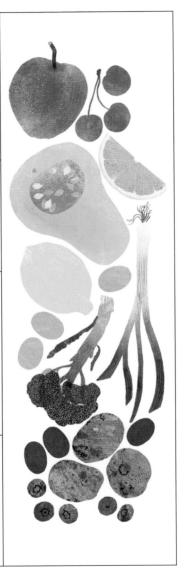

4. Sample a variety of flavours

When we don't eat all of the variety of flavours with each meal – salty, sweet, bitter, pungent and savoury – we may come away feeling like we are 'missing something', and food cravings can result. By getting small amounts of all the flavours of food, a practice common in other cultures, such as those of Japan, we may feel more fulfilled and desire less food after a meal. Using fresh herbs or spices is an excellent way to add flavour but also nutrients to your food. For example:

* Parsley is an excellent source of vitamins C and A

* Dill is rich in phytochemicals thought to support the immune system and cardiovascular health

* Cardamom, caraway seeds and aniseed can improve digestion and absorption of nutrients from the food they are cooked with

* Thyme and rosemary are thought to support respiratory health and brain function

5. Drink in between meals

Although keeping hydrated is key (and dehydration can often be mistaken as hunger or low energy), gulping liquid during meals can dilute the digestive enzymes needed to break down food and can lead to digestive problems. It's not that you shouldn't drink at all with food, but that reducing the amount you drink will support rather than hinder the digestive process. It's best to leave the majority of your hydration to in between meals.

6. Eat protein with every meal

Protein is needed to carry nutrients from food around the body. Protein also supports blood sugar balance and the repair of everyday wear and tear in the body. Protein sources are not only poultry, fish and lean red meats, but also nuts, seeds and pulses. Aim for 2–3 portions of protein per day. For guidance, a portion is a serving of meat the size of your fist – 120g of cooked pulses, 20g of nuts or seeds or 80g of tofu, for example.

VEGANS AND VEGETARIANS

The same principles apply to anyone following a vegan or vegetarian diet but eating a wider variety of protein, or 'protein combining', becomes even more important because plant-based protein sources are incomplete, meaning they lack certain essential amino acids. Choose alternative dairy sources such as natural soya and sources of healthy omega 3 fatty acids, such as walnuts or linseeds. Supplements that contain vitamin D, vitamin B12 and iron are often an important support too.

7. Choose nourishing carbohydrates

Replace non-nourishing carbohydrates with nourishing carbohydrates (see opposite) that will nourish your body and balance your energy levels and weight. Aim for 3–4 portions of nourishing carbohydrates (each portion is around one handful of cooked grains). Fruit and vegetables are also good sources of carbohydrates, so these can be counted as sources too.

Non-nourishing carbohydrates	Nourishing Carbohydrates
Refined white flour – white bread, packaged cereals, cakes, puddings, pastries & biscuits, white pasta	Wholegrains – wholemeal flour, wholegrain pasta, barley, millet, spelt, quinoa, brown rice, buckwheat, rye flour, porridge oats
Refined white sugar – sweets, chocolate, jams/marmalades, golden syrup, glucose, fizzy drinks Artificial sweeteners	Unrefined sugars – demerara sugar, honey (manuka or local untreated variety), black treacle, raw and organic dried fruit, maple syrup

8. Don't forget healthy fats

Healthy fats within your meals are important too and without enough of them our bodies and minds can begin to suffer. You need only a small amount (about 10 per cent of your meal) but enriching your meals with foods rich in healthy fats including nuts, seeds, avocados, cold-pressed virgin olive oil and full-fat yoghurt can go a long way in supporting your overall wellbeing. Avoid cooking with cooking oils where you can, instead adding them to food once cooked.

9. Eat regularly but not too often

Modern research is showing us that having fasting breaks between meals and avoiding snacking has many health benefits, including balanced energy and helping to prevent inflammatory conditions later in life. I have seen the benefits of this for those I have worked with too. Fasting windows of 12–16 hours overnight, so that we are eating our meals within an 8-hour window, appear to offer the greatest benefits. However, it is very important to remember that these sustainable and long-term benefits come only when we are eating properly balanced and nourishing meals when we do eat, by building in the principles discussed here. Starting the day well is especially important, reducing cravings later in the day when our energy or blood sugar levels drop. It's also worth remembering that although this is supported by modern research, it is very much replicating the way in which our ancestors ate.

There are some exceptions to this guideline – for children and for pregnant or breastfeeding women, for example – so look out for this advice in Parts Two and Three.

10. Keep active

Exercise, like food and eating, can be a confusing and divisive topic, with some championing the benefits of high intensity workouts while others campaign for less intensity and more stretching. I am not a sports scientist and I do not wish to advocate one route or another but what I can say is that movement matters, every day.

Public Health England recommend all adults aged 16–64 take part in at least 150 minutes of moderate intensity exercise or 75 minutes of vigorous activity (these can be broken down into 10- or 15-minute chunks), or a mixture of the two, each week. Additionally, it is recommended that all adults take part in muscle- strengthening activities, such as weight lifting or yoga, every week as well.

You can also make small changes to your non-exercise activity thermogenesis (NEAT) output. NEAT is the energy expended by our bodies when were awake (but doesn't include when we are eating or exercising) and there are simple things that you can do to increase this, such as carrying bags of shopping, walking rather than using the car or taking the stairs instead of the lift. Domestic activity that is part of your day-to-day life, such as window washing or hoovering, all contributes too.

Exercising in nature as much as possible can be hugely beneficial to our health too – exercising in green areas has been shown to reduce stress and improve mood and self-esteem more than exercising indoors. From my experience, it can help us feel more grounded and connected to our environment too. So, where you can, exercise outdoors, whatever the weather.

But it is the power in the relationship between the food we eat and exercise that will make the difference. As Henry Dimbleby writes in his book *Ravenous: How to Get Ourselves and Our Planet into Shape*, you can't outrun a bad diet.

There are also some easy tips you can incorporate into your cooking and shopping practices.

11. Prioritise sleep

Most of us know how nourishing sleep can be but not all of us put that into action. Many natural therapists and indeed doctors might feel that half their job is already done if they could sell sleep to their patients and clients! It's Mother Nature's natural healer and should be valued just as much as eating well. You will find some simple ways to support the quality of your sleep on pages 106–09.

Preparing food

Every mealtime, we can make choices about how we want to nourish ourselves, through the foods we eat but also the way that we cook them. It is also an opportunity for a mindful, creative practice at the end of day or to look after ourselves or others, or in advance of a busy week with a day of batch cooking.

Just by preparing and cooking meals yourself, you are benefiting your health, simply because you are unlikely to use the same number of artificial flavours, preservatives, sugar, salts or damaging fats that are included in many pre-prepared foods. Cooking for yourself means you have the chance to choose nutrient-dense ingredients such as wholegrains rather than refined grains, for example. One study found that those who ate five or more homecooked meals a week (breakfast, lunch or dinner) were 28 per cent less likely to be overweight than those who ate three or less. So, while there will be times we may need to lean on prepared meals or takeaways, cooking from scratch whenever possible can make a big difference to our health.

The way that you shop for, prepare and cook your food can help you to maximise nutritious eating.

Fruit and vegetables

* Shopping for fresh fruit and vegetables two or three times a week is better than making one big purchase because they lose their nutrient value fairly quickly as they age, so keeping them as fresh as possible can make a difference. When fruit becomes too 'soft' the fruit 'sugars' increase, so try to eat fruit at its peak of ripeness.

* When it isn't possible to buy fresh fruit and vegetables, opt for frozen rather than tinned. Though some frozen foods, such as peas and berries, contain comparable nutrient levels to the fresh variety, others, such as broccoli and beans, do not, so try to buy these fresh when you can.

* Once fruit and vegetables are cut, they start to lose their nutrient content. Chop them only when you are ready to cook them, if possible.

* Rather than throwing away the stems of vegetables such as broccoli, use them in soups and juices or grate them into cooking because they are packed with nutrients and far too good to waste!

Cooking

Cooking for yourself can be just as speedy and convenient as buying a prepared meal, with some very nourishing meals ready within 15 minutes (think wholemeal pasta with a homemade pesto of fresh kale, Parmesan and cashew nuts, for example).

*   Steaming rather than boiling helps food to retain its nutrients, whereas boiling causes the nutrients to leach into the water. If you do boil, use as little water as possible and save this water to use in soups and sauces.

*   Quick frying or roasting with olive oil has less of an impact on the protein or mineral content of potatoes than deep-frying or using sunflower oil.

*   Boiling potatoes with their skins on reduces the nutrient value lost when compared to peeled, but baking and steaming offer the most health benefits.

*   Keeping the skin on your vegetables or fruit can also affect its nutrient value. For most fruit and vegetables, the nutrients are stored just under the zest and the skins are also a great source of fibre. However, conventionally grown fruits and vegetables can retain chemical sprays or are bleach-washed prior to reaching our shelves. If you choose non-organic produce, consider using a vegetable wash (you can buy these or make your own with baking soda) instead of peeling them. If you chose organic varieties, or those sourced from places where you know sprays are not used, scrub them and cook them with their skins on.

The ripple effect

By rediscovering or furthering your passion for real food, you also have the potential to be a positive influence on those around you too. This is especially important if you have children. They may not adopt these processes immediately, especially if you have teenage children, but by osmosis this positive attitude will sink in.

The state of the global food industry may be bleak, but with an increased knowledge of nutrition and how to get the most from your food, you can still provide your body with the nourishing foundations needed for a healthy future. By eating locally sourced, seasonal food and by taking the recommended supplements, you can improve your own wellbeing.

Our spiritual relationship with health and food

We have as much, or arguably more, to learn about eating and food from history, culture and tradition as we do from science. Our separation from the wisdom and ceremony of food in recent generations has meant that we have lost a lot of the heart and soul which goes into the food cycle, commoditising our food and being too short on time to celebrate and share it.

It is the culture of eating and its role in ritual, ceremony and spiritualism that we need to resurface. It is a form of love and nourishment, for ourselves and for others, but wholesome food cultures and practices don't just happen, they are made by us. We can reactivate this in our communities – whether that is in a community of one, our family home, in our workplace or local community.

Food is at the nexus of healthcare and of spiritual, emotional, mental and planetary wellbeing. In *Soil, Soul and Society*, environmental activist Satish Kumar elucidates Eastern wisdom for the West, reminding us that caring for the natural environment (soil), maintaining personal wellness (soul) and upholding human values (society) are the moral imperatives of our time. To address mental and physical health, planetary health and spiritual health, therefore, we have to respect the interwoven nature of all these strands; it is a question of unification rather than separation.

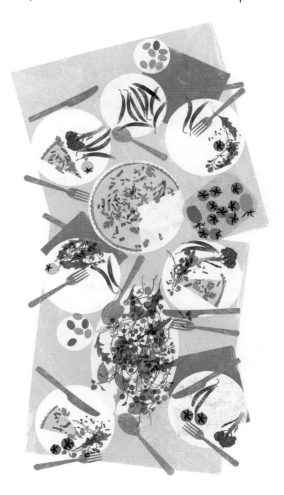

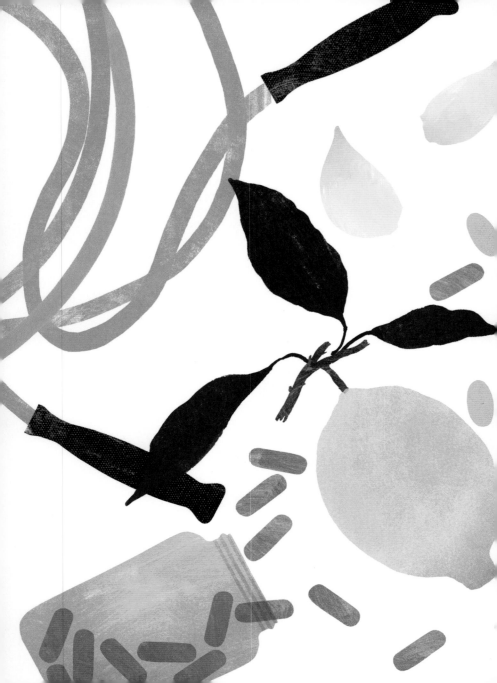

PART TWO

Maximising Health at Every Age

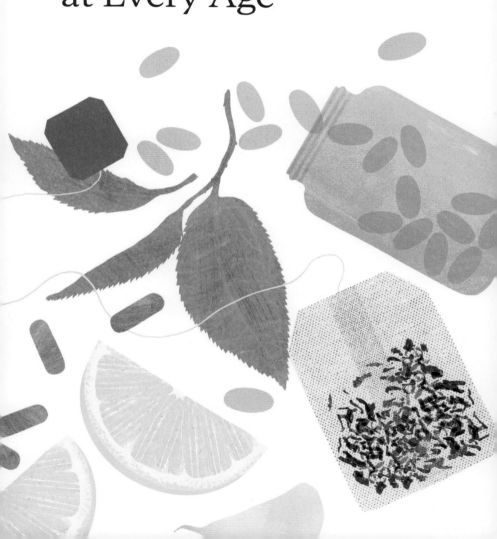

INTRODUCTION

Our bodies are miraculous, quite a triumph of Mother Nature. Each of us is a system of 206 bones, 100 trillion cells and 90,000 miles of nerves passing signals from head to toe. We all experience times when we realise how wildly complex our body really is, and that it needs the right nutritional support to carry us through – whether it is pregnancy, illness, ageing or simply moving into a different life stage. Our health is our own journey and our needs often change, depending on the stage of life we are in, our sex or the life circumstances around us.

In this section of the book, we will look at the differing needs at various stages, how to support ourselves through nutrition and holistic lifestyle interventions, and when we might need to turn to supplements to bridge the gap. All the recommendations made in this section are in addition to the Natural Wellbeing Foundations on pages 29–39. These really are the essential building blocks on which to further a positive relationship with our health, and remain essential, no matter what stage of life you are in.

The supplement recommendations I make are for naturally-sourced supplements, which deliver nutrients in a form that your body can assimilate easily and that respect the intelligence of the body. This may also mean that some of the doses I recommend are lower (because of the superior absorption) than you may see elsewhere.

BIRTH TO EARLY PUBERTY

The period between birth and early puberty is one of the most challenging times of our lives. Growth is rapid and the demand on our body is incredible.

Infancy: 0–12 months

The stage directly after birth is often known as the fourth trimester. This is the time of greatest physical growth in our child's life. In fact, they won't grow again at this rate until they hit early adolescence. It is also a time of significant emotional growth and physical demand for us parents too, especially mothers, as we heal and restore our bodies from birth and (for some of us) during the subsequent breastfeeding. It is a miraculous and demanding stage of life for everyone and a time to focus on and meet your needs through a nourishing diet, rest and permission to take life more gently.

Perhaps the most fascinating of changes occurs in ways we can't see – in our baby's immune system. In the womb and during the birth process, babies begin to develop their immune system. This happens by a process of exchange, whereby the mother passes her antibodies to her baby via the placenta.

Over 70 per cent of our immune system as adults is found in the tissue within our gut. These immune cells communicate with, and are influenced by, the amount and diversity of bacteria in our gut, which plays a fundamental role in the development and adaptability of our immune system. And here is another example of the intelligence in nature: during a vaginal birth, the beneficial bacteria in a mother's vaginal canal is ingested by her baby on the way through, as a 'starter pack' for the baby's own gastro-centric immune system. This is then built on by more antibodies that are passed to the baby from the colostrum found in the early stages of breastfeeding. Over time, the baby builds up their own immune system through a combination of exposure to the environment, their mother's milk and, eventually, the vitamins, minerals and other nutrients in weaning foods.

It is well understood that the blueprint for our health is in development when we are in our mother's womb. Here, the foundations are laid and many important things – such as our vulnerability to stress as young children or our risk of cardiovascular disease as adults – are determined. But as we emerge into the outside world, we become increasingly dependent on our external environment to support our health and development.

In the first four to six months, a baby requires a hefty number of macronutrients: protein, fat and carbohydrate, in addition to the key essential micronutrients, including vitamin D, vitamin B12, vitamin A, vitamin C, calcium, iron and zinc.

In formula milk, these will be composed scientifically and carefully balanced.

If the baby is being breastfed, these nutrients will be enriching the breastmilk from the mother's diet. The only thing you may wish to add directly to the baby's diet is vitamin D, as explained opposite. Otherwise, it is the mother's nutrition we focus on during this period. In particular, a breastfeeding mother will need more calcium and vitamin B12 in her diet than she did when she was pregnant, and taking supplements in this period is well worth considering. For more information on which supplements may be beneficial, see pages 196–199.

Whether or not you are breastfeeding, though, a healthy diet is so important to support you post-pregnancy and birth. The right nutrients and adequate rest help to restore hormonal balance and replenish nutrient stores that have been diminished. Your immune system and energy levels are highly likely to be affected by disrupted sleep, so both parents taking care of their nutrition so that they can thrive and flourish during this time is really the best advice.

⬚ Supplements for 0–12 months old

Supplements are not required for a baby who is receiving over 500ml of formula milk that contains 400iu/10ug of vitamin D and is fortified with vitamins A and C. However, if your baby is breastfed, it is recommended that you supplement their diet with 8.5–10mcg of vitamin D.

Toddler and preschool: 1–4 years

This stage is less immediately dramatic in terms of growth than the first year, but within a relatively short period of time, it seems, our newborn has become a walking, talking toddler. Our child is acquiring new skeletal muscles and tissues, so it's an important time to make sure that they get all the calories from the right sources to power this growth.

Just like the physical body, the brain is developing rapidly, with billions of neuronal extensions being created, particularly between the ages of one and two, most of which are built from fats and proteins. So it's not surprising that the requirement for essential fatty acids, omega 3, are high in this stage of childhood. Right now, there's not a major difference between boys and girls in terms of their energy or nutrient needs.

The other headline nutrients that are in high demand are calcium, phosphorous, potassium and zinc. Deficiency in any one can hinder growth at this stage.

It is a UK government recommendation for children under the age of five years old to take a daily supplement that contains vitamins A, C and D (which is available free of charge for low-income families in the UK through the Healthy Start scheme). In an ideal world, children's diets would supply these key nutrients, but given the prevalence of picky eating in this age bracket, supplementation gives another level of assurance that your child is taking in the necessary amounts.

Vitamin A is important for healthy brain and eyesight development, among other functions. Vitamin C supports growing joints and aids the absorption of iron, alongside its better known role supporting the immune system, while vitamin D is crucial for brain and immune development.

This is the time when we can start to build good foundations with our child for a love of food and eating, not simply for the nutrients but also the ritual of eating meals at a table with others. But it is a demanding time for everyone, and any parent of an active toddler will have times – probably many times! – when they feel that certain nutritional needs aren't being met, whether this is due to their own hectic work-life balance, or a fussy eater. These blips in nutrition and rest are manageable if they are infrequent, but when they become chronic, as it can with many of us, we begin to run into depletion. Getting sufficient rest or time to nourish yourself properly is still vital at this stage (in fact, at any stage); see the foundations of a healthy diet on page 29 for ways to build up nutrition as a parent.

Supplements for toddlers and pre-schoolers

A multi-nutrient formulated for children: This will contain calcium, zinc, iron, vitamins D and A (or beta-carotene), which are also a key focus at this stage to support growth and brain development. During the weaning stage, iron deficiency is the most common nutrient deficiency in developed countries.

Good food sources of vitamin A and its precursor beta-carotene	Good food sources of vitamin C	Good food sources of vitamin D	Good food sources of iron
Dairy products	Tomatoes	Oily fish, such as salmon	Red meat (unprocessed)
Eggs	Peppers		
Carrots, squash, sweet potatoes	Broccoli	Dairy foods, such as milk and yoghurt	Pulses such as lentils and chickpeas
Peppers	Kale		Pumpkin Seeds
Dark green vegetables, such as spinach, kale and broccoli	Oranges		Spinach
	Kiwi fruit	Egg yolk	Quinoa
Pumpkin seeds and cashew nuts	Potatoes (including sweet potatoes)	Sunshine	Tofu
Fruits, including papaya, apricots and mangoes	Strawberries		

Schoolchildren: 5–12 years

Healthy girls and boys are expected to gain around 30cm in height and 12kg in weight between five and ten years old. Lymphatic tissue (a significant part of the immune system called the 'adaptive' immune system, which helps us to adapt to our environment) grows most rapidly during this stage, doubling in size between six and twelve years of age. Children need a range of micro- and macronutrients to keep up with the demands of this growth, as well as those of the active school day, but this is when nutritional needs start to vary more from child to child, according to a range of factors, such as physical activity level. Early signs of puberty can occur at this stage, with some girls reaching their pubertal growth spurt at eight, which affects nutritional requirements considerably. Iron, zinc and calcium are still key at this stage for the development of the brain and nervous system, though studies show that many children are significantly below the required intake of these vitamins.

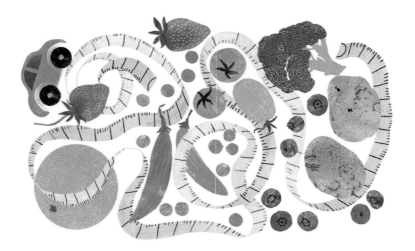

But life is not always simple and getting the right nutrients to support this growth can be more challenging. Not least because children begin to spend more time outside the family environment at this stage too, playing with peers, going to school and perhaps afterschool care, which lessens the opportunities to have a say in what they are eating away from home. They are also rapidly taking on the values and tastes of their peers and becoming susceptible to advertising, with advertisers exploiting this vulnerability.

The average child between two and twelve years of age old eats two pieces of fruit per day, though chocolate, biscuits, crisps, fish fingers, chips, cake and chicken nuggets appear in surveys as the top ten consumed foods. It's important to say here that a little of something here and there is no great shakes – I am a mother to three children myself and know all too well the attraction they hold – but it becomes an issue when these foods are the mainstay of the diet.

Here are some of the key nutritional areas to be aware of at this life stage:

Fats
This age group requires only a small amount of natural saturated or unsaturated fats, but it is important for children because it is rich in fat-soluble nutrients, including vitamin D for brain and immune development (as well as vitamin A for eye health).

Carbohydrates and fibre
For children at this age, half of their energy should be coming from unrefined carbohydrates such as wholegrains, which also provide the fibre they require at this stage too (20g per day). The rest should be made of natural proteins needed for developing muscles and tissues as they grow.

Vitamin C
This is important to maintain a healthy immune system, as well as for building connective tissue around growing joints and wound healing. I can remember the early school years as a hothouse for bugs, flus and scrapes from playground tumbles, so ensuring you are topping up vitamin C levels is key. Signs of deficiency can be recurrent colds and flus, bleeding gums, easy bruising of the skin or poor wound healing. It also works to aid the absorption of iron, another key nutrient for healthy growth at this stage. In nature, they are often found together, along with vitamin B2. The NRV for vitamin C is 60mg and the requirement for children below 12 years of age is 50 per cent of this, so 30mg.

Easy ways to get more vitamin C into their diet which are likely to go down well include making tomato soups or blackberry compotes during the autumn or winter season, chopping parsley into cooked food or making smoothies with a mixture of kale and kiwi fruit. It is helpful to be aware that boiling vegetables can leach the vitamin C into the water, so either steam or use the cooking water for soups or stews. See page 51 for some good sources of vitamin C.

Vitamin A
This is important for healthy brain and eyesight development, as well as immunity and healthy skin, helping to protect your child from playground sniffles as well as promoting growth. Dry skin, including eczema, slow wound healing, regular throat or chest infections or delayed growth are all signs of possible vitamin A deficiency. Beta-carotene and the carotenoid group of plant chemicals generate retinol, a potent form of vitamin A, when we eat them. Therefore, eating foods rich in these can really help. The NRV for vitamin A is 800ug and the requirement for children below 12 years of age is 50 per cent of this, so 400ug.

Setting up children for success with good food habits can have a measurable impact on their relationship with food and health into their adult years. It's important to remember that they are attuned to our habits and behaviours at this point. So, while the idea of helping children to develop lasting healthy habits may seem daunting, one of the main things we can do is to set them the example that meals are a point of pleasure and communication, and to show our love of food, not a fear or disregard for it. It can also be an opportunity, or a ritual, for us to connect with our children at the end of their day.

Early childhood is an important time for children to try new foods and develop good habits and healthy behaviour. Conflicts over meals is normal and, usually, transient. Young children should not be force-fed if refusing. It is best to make mealtimes happy and relaxed. Continue to introduce new foods, as well as reintroducing those that have been refused in the past – research has found that children who tried a vegetable that they didn't like began to like it more after the eighth time of trying it. So often it comes down to perseverance and patience. Below are some food hacks to get more nutrients into the diet of children in this age group (and sometimes older ones too!).

Food hacks for picky eaters

Always be on the lookout for creative ways with which to subtly reintroduce foods they have turned their nose up at, such as grating vegetables into sauces. Grating carrots or puréeing peppers and adding into tomato sauce to use on pasta is a great way of creating a more nourishing meal.

Stewed fruit with cinnamon or nutmeg can be a great way to build in more fruit – save them in ice-cube trays and defrost as you need to add to yoghurt or porridge. (But bear in mind that there will be a high sugar content, so limit portion size.)

Frozen fruit and vegetables can contain just as many nutrients as fresh and are quick and easy to prepare. They can also be good low-cost alternatives and can help to reduce waste because you tend to use only what you need. You can add frozen vegetables to pasta sauces, soups, stews, stir-fries and curries, and use frozen fruit in smoothies (maximum of 150ml of smoothie a day) or defrost them to use on top of plain yoghurt or porridge.

Some meals (such as cottage or fish pie and Bolognese sauce) freeze well, so when you do have time, consider doubling quantities of dishes that are popular with the whole family and freezing in meal-sized packs for a quick dinner when time is short. This makes it less likely you will have to resort to less healthy alternatives.

Invest in a slow cooker – this is a great way to save time and still prepare a healthy meal. If you can make time for some prep in the morning when your baby is having a nap or the kids are at school, putting the ingredients in the slow cooker, then at end of the day, dinner is ready. Just like that.

Supplements for schoolchildren: 5–12

A multi-nutrient formulated for children: This is especially important if you have a child who doesn't eat a wide variety of foods or has a low appetite. Look for formulas that provide iodine, vitamin D, iron, beta-carotene (or vitamin A).

Vitamin D: For children from the age of one, 400iu of vitamin D is recommended per day. So if this is not in your child's multi-nutrient, consider adding it in as a separate supplement.

Omega 3 supplement: Research has shown that the majority of young children are not getting sufficient omega 3-rich foods into their diet. Look for a supplement that has a ratio of 2:1 DHA to EPA and provides at least 250mg of DHA (see below for more on this). Choose a supplement from a sustainable source with good traceability and purity.

THE PURITY OF OMEGA OILS: WHAT ARE EPA AND DHA?
EPA and DHA are two types of the fatty acids also known as omega 3 fats.
Eicosapentaenoic acid (EPA): This is used by the body to produce a group of chemicals within the immune system known as eicosanoids, which in turn help to control inflammation. EPA may also help reduce symptoms of depression and support a balanced mood.

Docosahexaenoic acid (DHA): This makes up about 8 per cent of brain weight and contributes to brain development and function.

A third type of omega 3 fatty acid is called **alpha-linolenic acid (ALA)**. It is found in plant and seed oils and needs to be converted by the body into EPA and DHA. However, this conversion can be inefficient and therefore direct sources of DHA and EPA are often chosen.

ADOLESCENCE: 12–19 YEARS

I don't think many of us would say now that we loved being a teenager. And it's not always a picnic for those around them, either. They will see their bodies go through physical changes, while hormones fluctuate with greater force and bring emotional and mental changes, as well as changes to skin and the start of menstruation. Changes to their brain, specifically a section called the amygdala, mean that they may be more sensitive and reactive to people around them and their environment. They may interpret our faces differently, hearing firm voices as shouting or straight faces as anger. Teenagers often get flak from those around them for being lazy or moody. While adults – particularly women – have had time to get used to the effect of their own hormones, teenagers are navigating this stage in the dark, having never been here before. For first-time parents, you are too. It can be overwhelming and although the temptation is to spend most of these years frustrated and cross with our teenage children, it is a time for compassion and support.

It is also a time when we start to see developmental and nutritional differences in boys and girls, and when puberty, for many, begins, although hormonal growth spurts for girls typically start two years earlier than with boys. Menarche in girls generally occurs between 12 and 13½ years of age. This can be determined by the mother's menarche age but also environmental influences, such as physical activity, weight and nutrition.

Stress and pressure can increase at school and socially, and yet the hormonal changes and adaptions occurring in the brain have been shown to make concentration even more difficult for young people at this stage. It has always puzzled me why we put the most academic pressure on our children at a time when they are perhaps challenged the most developmentally. This is compounded by the shift in their circadian rhythms, which means that their bodies naturally favour going to bed late and getting up late, which can be at odds with the typical school day. Adequate rest is a key foundation stone for healthy growth and development at this stage, though enforcing that can be challenging!

Adolescents comprise 20 per cent of the world's population and yet, it seems to me, are greatly underserved in the area of health and nutrition in comparison to childhood years. Growth and development is rapid during these years and the demand for almost all nutrients is higher. The key ones to be aware of at this stage are iron, zinc and calcium.

Iron
Girls can lose an average 44ml of blood from menstruation every four weeks. This is equivalent to a loss of 12.5umol blood iron per day. This is why the need for iron in girls at this stage increases, though, according to the British Nutrition Foundation, almost 50 per cent of teenage girls do not get enough in their diet.

It is important to note that iron is needed by both girls and boys to support energy and cognitive health. It is also key for making red blood cells, which carry oxygen around the body.

Good sources of iron are:

* red meat and liver

* wholegrains (such as wholemeal bread)

* iron-fortified breakfast cereals

* dark green vegetables (such as kale, watercress)

* beans (such as red kidney beans, chickpeas)

* dried fruits (such as figs, raisins) and seeds (such as sesame seeds, pumpkin seeds)

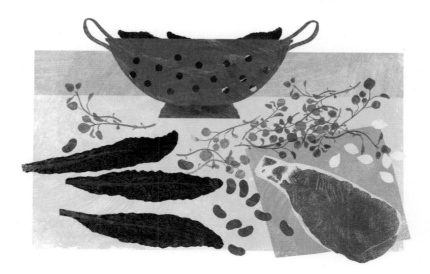

These foods also tend to be high in folate – a water-soluble natural B vitamin and another nutrient needed for growth and brain development.

Tea and coffee contain polyphenols (plant compounds) which can bind to iron and reduce how much of it is absorbed into the body, so try to avoid drinking them with your meals.

GOOD SOURCES OF IRON FOR VEGANS AND VEGETARIANS

- Pulses (lentils, beans and peas)

- Green leafy vegetables (such as watercress and spinach)

- Wholemeal bread

- Some fortified breakfast cereals (with added iron)

- Dried fruits (such as apricots and figs)

- Nuts and seeds (such as cashews, almonds, walnuts, sesame seeds, pumpkin seeds and sunflower seeds)

Iron found in plant foods is less readily absorbed than that from animal products like meat and eggs. However, vitamin C can help your body to absorb iron from plant sources, so try to combine foods or drinks high in vitamin C with those containing iron. Vitamin C-rich vegetables include broccoli, kale, Brussels sprouts, cabbage, peppers and tomatoes.

Calcium

There is a significant change to a teenager's skeleton too, going through the most rapid change of any life stage. In boys, the skeletal growth spurt is greater than in girls and is accompanied by accelerated muscle growth, meaning that boys' requirements rapidly diverge from those of girls. This is where peak bone mass is acquired for boys – in fact, over 25 per cent of total bone mass is acquired during this stage and into early adulthood, where it will be 25–30 per cent greater than that of young men. This seismic drive of skeletal growth increases the body's demand for calcium (for boys, it is nearly double the amount than needed in childhood) – as well as phosphorous, magnesium and vitamin D. This greater demand falls again after the age of 19, but up until that point a supplement programme to provide enough of these minerals is essential.

Good sources of calcium are:

* dairy products, such as milk, yoghurt and cheese

* calcium-fortified dairy alternatives (particularly important if you are vegan or do not eat dairy products)

* almonds

* dark green vegetables (such as kale, rocket and watercress)

* fish that is eaten with the bones (such as whitebait, canned sardines or canned salmon)

Physical activity is also an influence on the increase in bone density in adolescence. It is thought that optimising bone health in early life might delay the onset of osteoporosis later. As teenagers are famed – and I have personal evidence of this also – for being sofa or bed surfers, gentle encouragement to be active, and preferably outside, is important for mental as well as physical health, and of course vitamin D exposure too.

Zinc

The hormonal shifts that come with the onset of puberty bring changes in weight, in mood and, for some, in skin, with the development of acne or spots. Research has shown that nutrient deficiencies in zinc and vitamin A, as well as imbalances in gut flora, can influence the development or inhibit repair from skin conditions such as acne or eczema. See page 96 for advice on managing acne and 96–7 for advice on eczema.

Teenagers can put their body under a microscope, scrutinising how it looks to themselves but also to those around them. One report showed that over half of teenage girls and nearly one third of teenage boys use unhealthy weight control behaviours, such as skipping meals, fasting, smoking cigarettes, vomiting and taking laxatives (Neumark-Sztainer, 2011). It's also important to note that teenagers will easily swing between over- and under-eating, and this affects intake of nutritionally supportive foods. This is harder for us to monitor, what with the power of influencers on social media, who are often peddling unfounded and unhealthy techniques.

Changes in hormones combined with more access to stimulants such as coffee, energy drinks and sweeter foods (that may have been previously limited by parents) may give way to blood sugar fluctuations.

What is blood sugar balance?

Your body is reliant on a steady amount of glucose being available in your blood. This is primarily controlled by a hormone that you may have heard of called insulin, which is produced in your pancreas. Its role is to take away excess sugar from the blood and store it in your fat cells. This helps to keep your blood glucose levels steady. However, a glucose 'high' is often followed by a glucose 'low', and it is this yo-yoing that makes us feel unwell and can cause longer term health issues, such as insulin resistance and diabetes. The foods that we eat and the times that we eat them can determine how steady or up-and-down our blood glucose levels are, but so can our stress levels and hormones such as oestrogen. Foods and drinks high in sugar, caffeine, trans fats or, importantly, foods stripped of fibre and protein, spike our blood glucose levels, whereas wholegrains, lean proteins and naturally fibre-rich foods steady our blood glucose levels. Signs of erratic or yo-yoing blood glucose levels are:

* Irritability, especially before (feeling hangry!) or after eating
* Anxiety or heart palpitations
* Depression and mood swings
* Poor concentration/brain fog
* Feeling easily stressed
* Storing fat around the middle of your body
* Waking in the night/fitful sleeping
* Poor energy unless after eating or drinking something with coffee or sugar
* Craving caffeine or sweet foods and emotional eating
* Regularly feeling thirsty despite drinking 1–1.5 litres of water
* Sweating easily, not related to exercise

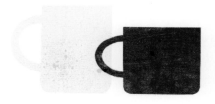

Nutrition for teenagers

Getting the right nutrients, in the right quantities can present a challenge for parents and adolescents, as our teenagers gain more autonomy over their food choices, often eating at least one meal (and plenty of snacking in between) outside of their homes. Additionally, you are fighting nature, as during times of stress (and this includes physiological stress from intense periods of growth) our bodies and brains are wired to seek out energy-dense foods. In times gone by, this would have been through more grains, potatoes and meat, but nowadays, it's the brightly coloured junk foods that tend to catch their attention and appetites. Teenagers are sitting ducks for advertisers and it is no wonder that this age group is increasingly the target demographic for energy drinks, and high-fat and high-sugar products, many of which are purposely priced to be accessible. These foods have negative effects for many reasons. If this is what teenagers are filling themselves with during the day, they may not have the appetite for a home-cooked meal at the end of it.

Food high in sugar and salt can change their taste buds too, which lose their sensitivity to naturally sweet or salty foods. These foods are also known as anti-nutrients, which means that they can either block the absorption of nutrients and/or use up important nutrients to break these foods down into waste products. A rule of thumb we have had in our house, and one that I recommend to many, is to make two meals a day homemade, with one of them being breakfast. Having two well-balanced meals a day can go a long way to a well-balanced diet, despite what goes on in between these meals. Having nutritious snacks in the house, such as oatcakes and nut butters, for grab-and-go teenagers is also helpful. Nagging is unlikely to get you far, but identifying their favourite healthy snack and making sure it is in their eyeline when they open the cupboard is a good way to encourage positive habits.

Eat enough protein

This macronutrient needs to be the foundation for each meal – the amino acids found in protein are vital for muscle and brain development. Together with fats, they form the backbone of many hormones and brain chemicals that help to stabilise mood and energy. Boys need on average 52g of protein a day and girls need 46g. To give you an idea of what this looks like, this daily requirement could be fulfilled by, for example, two medium eggs and half a cup of pumpkin seeds, or 75g of cooked chicken, or one small piece of salmon (100g). Foods rich in protein tend to be rich in phosphorous too, which is needed for bone health.

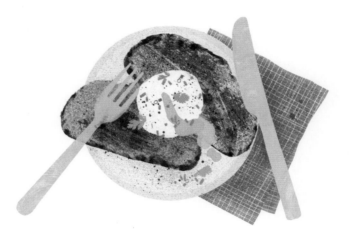

A good breakfast is the best start to the day

Build a breakfast based on protein, such as scrambled or poached egg on a piece of wholemeal bread, or a bowl of yoghurt with chopped fruit and nuts. Alternatively, a protein-based smoothie using yoghurt, a nut butter such as almond butter or a handful of nuts or seeds as the base ingredient will boost their intake of protein, fat and nutrients for the day ahead.

Think in rainbows
Getting as much colour into your diet is vital at all stages. For teenagers, plant chemicals or phytochemicals including polyphenols and carotenoids are particularly useful when they are stressed (or staying up far too late!) for supporting the immune system, brain development and muscle repair. Carotenoids are used by our body to generate vitamin A and this is especially important for skin health. Teenagers eat 2.9 portions of fruit and vegetables a day on average, below the recommended five – again, smoothies can increase this (though remember a maximum of 150ml) and soups too.

Don't forget the good fats
The group of fats named omega 3 is essential for healthy brain development and hormone balance. A deficiency has been associated with many health conditions and symptoms of ADHD, as well as impacting learning (Chang et al., 2019). Excellent sources of these are oily fish (sardines, mackerel, anchovies, salmon and herrings), eggs, and unsalted and unroasted nuts or seeds. Sprinkle a dessertspoon of mixed nuts or seeds into yoghurt, on porridge or use as a snack. Use oily fish to make fishcakes.

Get quality rest!
Teens need a minimum of eight hours sleep a night. Tips for better sleep include screen-free bedrooms, screen-free time before going to sleep and finding a relaxing routine before bed that works for them. Again, I know only too well that this can be a potential battleground, but this is where encouraging teenagers to engage with their own wellbeing and understand how rest and nutrition can help them in areas that interest them – such as giving them more energy to play sport, better skin or even improved grades – can set them up for the future and avoid descending into a nag cycle!

Supplements for teenagers

A good-quality multi-nutrient for teenagers: Check that they include iron (at least 7mg of iron for teen girls), zinc, vitamin B6 to support hormonal balance and the immune system, vitamin D, calcium for healthy bone development, and vitamins C, B12, B2, B1 and magnesium, which all support a normal energy.

Calcium: is important for both boys and girls and building calcium-rich foods into their diets as well as through supplementation is important. See pages 60–1 for more on calcium.

Omega 3 supplement: Preferably in a ratio of 2:1 EPA to DHA. (See pages 56–7 for more on this.)

Because of the stresses that can occur at this life stage, I often recommend plant adaptogens in supplement form for teenagers too. Adaptogens include mushrooms such as reishi and the ayurvedic herb ashwagandha, which contain properties traditionally used to fortify the body during times of growth and stress. Take these either on their own or within a supplement formulation.

See Part Three for supplements to support specific concerns, such as acne or hormonal issues.

WHAT ARE ADAPTOGENS?

Adaptogens are a group of plants, herbs and medicinal mushrooms that have the properties to help our bodies manage stress and restore balance after and during stress (from psychological or emotional stress but also physical stress such as injury). Some of my favourite adaptogens are:

Ashwagandha: an Ayurvedic herb to help reduce anxiety and depression.

Reishi and many of the other medicinal mushrooms commonly used in traditional Chinese medicine to support immunity, energy and resilience.

Tulsi or 'holy basil': another Ayurvedic herb to support anxiety, the immune system and focus.

There are many adaptogens available, and with so many of us feeling overstretched or stressed in some way, what is not to love about this group of natural stress supporters? I regularly recommend them throughout the different life stages.

YOUNG ADULTHOOD
TO MIDDLE YEARS

Although growth has slowed down significantly and therefore nutrient demand remains pretty consistent, this life stage can be one of increasing work demands, socialising and, in the early adult years, our first foray into living and cooking independently. Later, we may have families to care for or other people to support, and the demands on our time become more complicated. It can also be a time when we de-prioritise our connection to our body and wellbeing in favour of productivity.

At various times and for different reasons, we may find ourselves making food choices that are less nourishing (for example, due to a tight budget, lack of cooking skills, time pressures). Stress, inadequate quality sleep and greater access to alcohol are other contributory factors to less nutrition going in, but more energy needed going out.

The years of early adulthood can be our first introduction to living independently – moving out of home for university, college, travel or work. All of which can be both liberating and potentially overwhelming, and at these times, healthy eating and home cooking may not be the first priority. For most, it is making the pennies stretch as far as they can and/or socialising. We've all been young and I can certainly remember what it feels like to burn the candle at both ends.

Eating well is a life skill that, in times gone by, would be slowly built from childhood – helping to prepare or cook meals (in some cultures, this is happily still the norm) and essentially developing a relationship with and love of good food. However, for various reasons, many children reach young adulthood without having been engaged in meal preparation on a regular basis. So, it can come as quite a shock to be solely responsible for eating a balanced, well-prepared meal three times a day.

As we know, making sure you get the right balance of macro- and micronutrients is also important for long-term health, including our emotional and psychological health, both of which can feel more challenged when demands and responsibility seem comparatively high. At these times, the temptation to choose cheap, fast food over homecooked food is higher, tapping into our natural urge for instant gratification. When we are busy and stressed – as we will sometimes be, in the course of normal adulthood! – we can overlook the impact that food and drink have on our body and mind (and therefore our performance at work or studies).

Apart from the impact on long-term health, regularly drinking alcohol beyond the maximum intake of 14 units spread throughout a week (one unit comprising 175ml of wine or one pint of beer – see note on blood sugar on pages 62–3) can affect mental wellness too. It may make you feel less stressed in the very short term, but it reduces quality sleep and mental focus, ultimately resulting in more stress. Relying on caffeine or energy drinks can be another way of getting through times of stress, or when energy in does not match energy out, but caffeine too has a negative impact on health and wellbeing if consumed in excess (above 400mg per day).

Energy is key at this life stage and with our busy modern lives, 'feeling tired' can be commonplace. As we progress beyond our young adult years, we will naturally start to notice that we don't bounce back quite so easily! As a twenty-something, a late night, overindulgence in food and alcohol or just generally packing a lot in can be recovered from relatively fast. Later, our bodies will start to remind us that we are not invincible after all. Or perhaps we find ourselves challenged by specific health issues, such as hormone imbalances or immunity problems. For many of us, this is when we take more notice of our body's needs, but it really is important at every age.

Your incredible body is making and repairing 3.8 million cells every second, as well as generating energy, metabolising hormones, fighting off exposure to pathogens and building blood cells, among many other essential functions. And at this stage in life, it may be needing to increase all of these to keep up with our busy lifestyles. These processes require nutrients to support energy production. Balancing the energy going into your body with the energy that is going out is your priority. Stress management and supplementation help to replenish lost nutrients through dietary gaps or a lifestyle that includes an excess of caffeine, cigarettes, sugar, alcohol or stress, all of which increase the body's demand for certain nutrients.

Health hacks for busy adults

There are many benefits to batch cooking and preparing food in advance, such as saving time and helping you stick to a new eating plan or more mindful diet. It is a reliable way to be organised, plan meals and have the right foods available. Making as much as you can when you do have the time to cook and freezing meals into individual portions is so helpful in avoiding junk or defaulting to a takeaway you don't even want.

Work out exactly what you need to buy, make a shopping list and stick to it. Budgeting is a big part of student and early career life, and for many of us later life too. Planning your meals at the end of the week for the week ahead will reduce the temptation to buy foods you don't need and may also help you to cut down on food waste and save money.

Beans and pulses are an excellent source of protein for energy and fibre for gut health. Adding ingredients like chickpeas, lentils and tofu to curries, pasta sauces and stir-fries will bulk them out, make them go further and contribute significantly to a balanced diet.

Freezing fruit and veg preserves nutrients and, in fact, some frozen vegetables can even give you more of certain nutrients than fresh versions: frozen peas contain nearly double the amount of calcium of fresh peas. Fresh fruit and veg can start to lose their nutrients as soon as they are picked and over the (often long) journey to our shelves, whereas produce from the freezer section will usually have been frozen as soon as it is picked. Broccoli florets, for instance, are blanched before being frozen, retaining more plant chemicals such as carotenoids than pre-cut fresh veg. It can also be cheaper than fresh and may stop unused food going to waste because you can use the exact amount you want when you want it, saving you money. So don't worry if you often find yourself relying on frozen veg.

An ideal breakfast includes a starchy food like oats or wholemeal toast with a protein source like nut butter, yoghurt or eggs. This will fill you up and may help avoid feelings of hunger mid-morning.

Supplements for early adulthood to middle years

A good quality multi-nutrient: One that has been formulated for your sex (those formulated for women will often have more iron in them to support monthly menstruation). This should also include vitamin B5, vitamin B6, calcium and magnesium which all support normal energy production.

Vitamin D: Government advice is that all adults should consider taking a daily vitamin D supplement containing 10mcg of vitamin D per day, especially during the autumn and winter months. It is challenging to get enough vitamin D through the food we eat, and very little vitamin D is produced in the skin in the regions north of 37 degrees latitude during the winter months. You may be able to find this in your multi-nutrient but if not, take an additional supplement.

⚗ Testing

A health practitioner can do a blood test to measure the amount of vitamin D within your system. Deficiency of vitamin D is defined as having a level of 50nmol/L or below. However, many experts argue that the optimum level should be higher than 75nmol/l and indeed closer to 100nmol/l, so supplementation is often needed.

THE BENEFITS OF NATURALLY SOURCED VITAMIN D

Vitamin D is essential for the body to form calcitriol (known as the form of vitamin D that actually does the donkey work). Calcitriol plays a crucial role in the normal function of many systems in the body, including the immune system and the musculoskeletal system, acting as an agent in the absorption of calcium. Research has also shown just how important it is for neurological development, fertility, menopause and autoimmune conditions.

However, synthetic forms of vitamin D do not provide calcitriol and the body must go through several steps to create it. These steps can be problematic for some people, especially if we are older or have a kidney or liver condition, and it can mean that much of the 'dose' of this form of vitamin D can remain unprocessed and therefore redundant – this may be why very high doses are often prescribed, to overcome this issue. Some studies have shown that the more natural Food-Grown® form of vitamin D produces the more active calcitriol.

A recent randomised, parallel clinical study undertaken by the University of Queensland, Australia, compared the bioavailability of synthetic vitamin D in tablet form, synthetic vitamin D in spray form and Food-Grown® vitamin D in capsule form and showed that, when compared to leading high-street vitamin D supplements in tablet form, the Food-Grown® vitamin D in capsules was 100 per cent more effectively absorbed. In addition, the Food-Grown® capsules maintained greater concentration in the bloodstream for longer than both the tablet and the spray, meaning that the body could retain and store it more effectively. This may be why these natural forms seem to be effective at low dose.

Omega 3 supplement: Preferably in a ratio of 2:1 EPA to DHA (see pages 56–7 for more on omega 3).

OMEGA 3 SUPPLEMENTS – TG OR ETHYL ESTER

Omega 3 oils are a rich source of essential fatty acids DHA and EPA. In the UK, sources of omega 3 are no longer readily eaten and can even be excluded by certain dietary practices, making supplementation necessary. DHA and EPA balance the action of mega 6 polyunsaturated fatty acids (found in vegetable oils) in the body. An imbalance of omega 3 has been shown to contribute to chronic health conditions, including those associated with chronic inflammation and autoimmune conditions, among many others.

Adaptogenic support: My favourite adaptogenic herb for this life stage is ashwagandha. It has been traditionally used to support our resilience to stress and more recent scientific studies have shown that a form of ashwagandha known as KSM-66 at a dose of 300mg twice daily can reduce stress and stress-related food cravings within eight weeks, and significantly improve sleep duration and quality within ten weeks. Medicinal mushrooms are also helpful, such as cordyceps and reishi, as they also provide antioxidant support. See the box on adaptogens on page 68 and the section about stress on pages 102–4, in Part Three, for more.

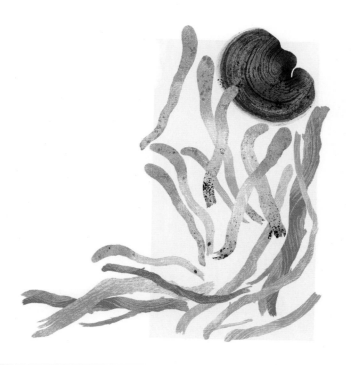

MIDDLE YEARS TO WISER YEARS

This life stage is an opportunity to age well, to engage with your health through diet, supplementation and activity that supports a vital health span. Life expectancy is over double that of the Victorian era, and according to the World Health Organisation, in 2050 it is estimated that over 2 billion of the world's population will be over 60. Yet despite the greater life span, we do not seem to be gaining a greater health span.

Interestingly, there is some crossover between our key nutritional needs at this later stage in our lives and what was important during puberty. For example, calcium is just as vital now to preserve our strong bones as it was when our bodies were growing them. Omega 3s were essential for brain development, and now they are central to brain protection.

Far from being a negative stage of life to fear, the period from our mid-forties onwards is a time when we can feel reconnected to ourselves and empowered to be an active part in our own self-care.

What is ageing?

Ageing is happening to us all, from birth. It is not something we can stop, despite a culture that encourages us to stay forever young. In fact, healthy ageing is something to be respected and valued. In traditional cultures, the elders of communities are revered for their wisdom and knowledge of traditional practices that will keep the communities well.

Scientifically speaking, ageing is a progressive decline in the efficiency of biochemical and physiological processes. It is thought, in part, to be predetermined in our genes; however, it is perhaps more greatly influenced by our exposure to oxidative stress.

Oxidative stress is, very simply, an imbalance between the rate at which we repair damage within the body cells and tissues – caused and restored by free radical and antioxidant processes respectively. Free radicals are oxygen-containing molecules that circulate around the body, borrowing electrons from other molecules and causing damage, whereas antioxidants are molecules that can donate an electron to the electron-seeking free radical without getting damaged themselves, thereby rendering the free radical more stable and less reactive. When there are more free radicals than antioxidants over a prolonged period of time, the rate of ageing or deterioration speeds up.

Oxidative stress is a natural internal process that is just par for the course. However, it is also caused by lifestyle factors such as environmental pollutants, nutrient-poor diets, diets high in sugar or trans fats, and stress. It can accumulate over our lifecycles and is associated with degenerative diseases including cardiovascular disease, cancer and neurodegenerative diseases. It can damage DNA, inhibit the 'repair' processes in the body and shorten telomeres (the 'shoelace caps' that protect cells from deterioration).

Natural changes occur in the competence of our immune system at this stage too. With a slow decline in the generation of lymphoid tissue, a significant part of our immune system, our response to and tolerance of infection is less robust, as is our ability to moderate inflammation. This can mean we are more prone to low-grade inflammation, which can speed up the ageing process and is now called 'inflammaging'. A growing body of research is showing us that inflammation is a root cause of many health risks at this life stage, including dementia, cancer, cardiovascular disease, arthritis and depression.

WHAT IS INFLAMMATION?

Inflammation is a protective mechanism that stimulates repair when we are ill, injured or exposed to environmental elements that the body deems threatening, such as stress or toxins. It is designed to be a short-term process that heals an area of damage or infection. However, today our bodies are exposed to more inflammatory triggers over a longer period, which creates chronic inflammation. Rather than being protective, this can have a negative effect and is associated with myriad health conditions, including cardiovascular disease, arthritis and depression, and also speeds up the ageing process.

We also know that, as we age, we become less responsive to vaccination against disease and that the most effective way to help our immune response is by paying attention to diet, nutrition and other principles of healthy living, such as supplementation, exercise and stress relief. When you look at it like this, taking the right supplements to ensure our needs are met looks far less like a luxury and much more like preventative care.

While there is no way to halt or reverse the natural ageing process, nutrition and lifestyle interventions have the potential to actively promote healthy ageing, reduce inflammaging and disease risk. How we eat and live has been shown to have a profound effect on the ageing process. This interaction between the way that we eat and our genes is known as nutrigenomics.

These middle years are when women experience significant hormonal shifts – the perimenopause and, finally, the menopause. Perimenopause is the period of time leading up to your final menstruation. It can last for a few months or several years. During this time, your periods may become irregular as your oestrogen and progesterone levels decrease – and you may experience menopausal symptoms. Post menopause is the time after menopause starting – from when you have not had a period for 12 consecutive months. See the section on perimenopause and menopause in Part Three, pages 175–83, for more on this, and particularly the effects of the fluctuating levels of oestrogen in the body.

Life changes for men too. Hormonal shifts, predominantly in testosterone, mean that men can experience an increase in fat mass, a decline in muscle mass and a change to cognitive health. This is called the andropause.

This stage of life for men and women can be mindfully managed with positive lifestyle factors, such as a good diet, supplements and appropriate activity. This can support immediate symptoms associated with the menopause and andropause and the inconveniences of ageing generally but also address some longer term health concerns, such as a higher risk of cardiovascular disease, osteoporosis and Alzheimer's.

Practising relaxation methods for just 10–20 minutes a day has been shown to activate genes that prevent cell ageing, control blood sugar and deactivate the genes responsible for chronic inflammation. Finding joy and regular laughter activates protective genes within the body which help repair cells and initiate healthy immunity – essential at a time when we are more prone to inflammation.

Activity levels at this life stage should be around 150 minutes spread over a one-week period and include weight-bearing activities for at least two sessions. Exercising outside and in company is the best approach: it will improve exposure to sunlight and therefore build up vitamin D, as well as supporting mood and sleep patterns.

Adequate sleep is crucial on a molecular level. Sleep deprivation can affect the activity of more than 700 genes, activating those involved in inflammation, immunity and protein damage and turning off those responsible for tissue regeneration. These changes occur when people sleep less than six hours a night.

Numerous studies have shown the benefit of eating a Mediterranean-style diet on the ageing process. Its natural richness in colourful plant foods, healthy oils and lean protein sources, such as fish, pulses and seeds, makes it the ideal foundation for healthy living and aligns with my health philosophy. It has been linked with lower mortality rates, reduced onset of multiple chronic diseases and improved cognitive function. In fact, one large study found that following a Mediterranean diet for one year improved the health of participants' microbiomes (see the section on digestion below), as well as significantly increasing levels of cytokines – substances released by the immune system to moderate inflammation.

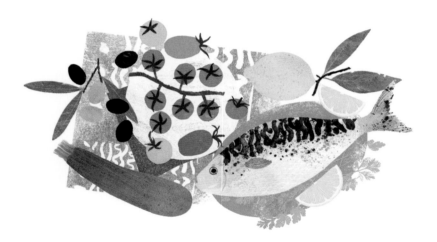

Good digestion

We are fast learning that good digestion is at the heart of good health. The gut is where we absorb nutrients, produce nutrients and serotonin, eliminate toxins and, to put it one way, empty our dustbin daily. Indeed, 70 per cent of the immune system is in the tissue of the gut and therefore it is pivotal in the moderation of inflammation.

However, it's important to know that our microbial diversity reduces with age, shifting more to an imbalance of less favourable than favourable bacteria and yeast (known as dysbiosis). Studies on centenarians show that the greater diversity of beneficial bacteria within the gut tissue (specifically bifidobacterium – a specific group of probiotic bacteria), the longer the life span. This may be because bifidobacterium species can actually reduce inflammation in places where it may be too high, and therefore reduce the negative impact it has on the rate of ageing.

The foods that form the cornerstone of the Mediterranean diet have been shown to promote good gut health, and epidemiological evidence also demonstrates that the longest living populations around the world often have a diet rich in fermented products – such as kimchi, sauerkraut, yoghurt, kefir – but also rich in colour and fibre. In these places, if meat is eaten, it is often slow-cooked to aid digestion.

How can we improve gut health for better ageing?

Eating a good mix of fruit and vegetables is always important, and particularly at this stage of life, not least because they are generally low in fat and high in fibre. Many studies have shown that people who consume diets high in fruit and vegetables have a lower risk of heart disease, stroke, diabetes and some forms of cancer. As rich sources of antioxidants, such as vitamin C and carotenoids, they can also help to counter the oxidative process of ageing.

Adults are recommended to have at least 30g of fibre daily. Average intakes are well below recommendations, with women managing only around 17g of dietary fibre per day. And while having a high-fibre diet may reduce the risk of heart disease, type 2 diabetes and bowel cancer at any age, this becomes especially relevant at this life stage when muscle tone naturally decreases and contractions in the gut, also known as peristaltic movement, can slow down. When waste matter becomes harder to excrete, it will remain in the gut for longer. Therefore, consuming enough fruit and veg can also support regular bowel movements and reduce the risk of constipation. A good thing to remember is to keep skins on vegetables and eat as wide a variety of colours of vegetables and fruit as possible each day.

Other key sources of dietary fibre are:

* Wholegrain and high-fibre varieties of starchy carbohydrates, such as wholegrain bread, wholewheat pasta, potatoes with skins on and high-fibre breakfast cereals

* Beans and pulses

* Nuts and seeds

As we age, our sense of taste, smell and strength of appetite can change. There is also a change in the number of digestive enzymes we produce, and therefore breaking down food and absorbing the nutrients from our food effectively can be harder.

Eating little and often and adding herbs and spices to your meals can increase the appeal, but it can also help with stimulating the right digestive juices to absorb food. For example, black pepper, ginger and fennel seeds can promote the production of salivary and digestive enzymes, whereas turmeric, cinnamon and fenugreek can help stabilise blood glucose levels after eating. Rosemary and turmeric have been used traditionally by those suffering inflammatory conditions and sage to support memory and brain function.

Experiment with textures of food as well so that the jaw can chew. Chewing stimulates the release of saliva and therefore the production of salivary enzymes for breaking down food.

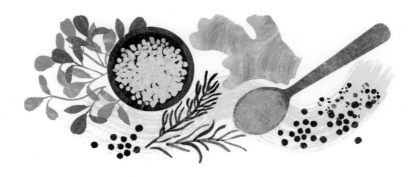

Protein

Healthy consumption of protein is also important. After the age
of around 30, we lose an average of 3–5 per cent of muscle every
decade, but at over 60 years of age, this rate increases. Protein is a
vital building block for healthy muscle generation and bone health,
making up a major part of the mass and volume, and creating a
meshwork of fibres that lay the foundation for growth – think of
protein as the scaffolding on which calcium and phosphorous then
form bone around.

Protein sources also provide a good supply of antioxidants and
amino acids, some of which increase cognition and improve heart
rate. Some amino acids – including NAC, acetyl-L-Carnitine, taurine,
methionine and cysteine – are also thought to have a positive impact
on protecting against degenerative diseases, including type 2 diabetes
and Alzheimer's, and even prematurely greying hair and hair loss.

However, as our bodies age, we become less efficient at
processing protein. So it is recommended to increase your protein
intake by 50 per cent after the age of 50, which means an average
of 82g for women and 97g for men. The best way of getting this
is through your diet, but reduced appetite can make this more
challenging than at other age stages. Therefore, supplementing with
a quality protein powder can be beneficial.

The importance of hydration

Water is vital for digestion, nutrient absorption, joint lubrication and temperature regulation. Not drinking enough water is common in older adults but it can contribute to several health problems, including increased risk of falls, constipation, urinary tract infections and cognitive impairment. Water and warm drinks such as herbal tea are obviously key, but also consuming hydrating foods, such as soups, fruits and vegetables can help to prevent dehydration, as well as ultimately supporting overall health and wellbeing.

Supplements for middle years to wiser years

As outlined in Part One, I am always an advocate for natural supplements because of their superior absorption, but I feel particularly strongly about championing the natural method of supplementation at this life stage when digestion can be poorer. The body's ability to absorb and utilise these natural nutrients is well documented and can make the difference to this age group being able to absorb the benefits or not.

A good quality multi-nutrient: As with all life stages, I recommend a good-quality, natural multi-nutrient tailored to suit this life stage, with at least 10mcg of vitamin D and 120mg of calcium.

Iron: Women up to the age of 50 years old continue to require more iron compared to men and older women. Iron is important for the development of red blood cells to help carry oxygen around the body but it is also essential for the immune system and the production of energy. Over a quarter of women aged 50 and below are estimated to have inadequate iron intakes and so the risk of iron deficiency anaemia is a little greater. Look for this as part of your multinutrient or take separately.

Omega 3 oils: Oestrogen is a cardio-protectant and therefore when oestrogen levels reduce as women get close to the menopause, our vulnerability to developing heart disease can increase with it (1 in 11 women die from heart disease). Omega 3 fatty acids are known to benefit cardiovascular as well as brain health for both men and women.

More recent research has also been looking at the role that these beneficial oils can have on other age-related conditions too, including rheumatoid arthritis and dementia. So, consciously including these in your diet at this life stage, through food and supplements, is very beneficial. A healthy diet should include at least one portion (140g cooked weight) of oily fish a week, but there are concerns about toxic metal pollution in these oilier fish, so it is recommended to eat no more than two portions per week.

Vitamin D: The body's ability to manufacture vitamin D3 from exposure to sunlight declines once we pass our sixties. At 70 years old, we produce only 25 per cent of the vitamin D made by a 20-year-old. Weight, sunscreen and high levels of atmospheric pollution can lower the generation of vitamin D from sunshine and food, but the greatest challenge for many at this life stage is getting sufficient time outside.

In 2021, researcher Sneha Baxi Srivastava suggested that exposure to sunlight for 5–15 minutes without sunscreen between the hours of 10am and 3pm during the spring, summer and autumn would be sufficient to improve vitamin D status. Getting out during daylight hours is great not only for vitamin D but also mood.

Vitamin D helps our bodies to absorb calcium (in the gut, which sends it to the bloodstream) and to regulate blood levels of calcium and phosphorus (which are needed to build bone, as I mentioned above). Vitamin D deficiency has been shown to increase the risk of fall and fracture in our older years, so for older people in particular, it is important to get levels checked annually, ideally in the autumn or winter.

Calcium: The rate at which we build and repair bone reduces as we age. This process of build and repair determines our bone density (how much bone mineral there is in the tissues in your bones). Therefore, loss of bone density is both natural and common as we get older, but we can control the rate at which this happens and therefore the risk of conditions such as osteoporosis. Calcium is a fundamental mineral for retaining this bone density and therefore it is key that we incorporate it into our diets as well as our supplement regimes. Oestrogen has a protective function over the rate at which bone is broken down and therefore women in the post-menopausal stage of life are at a higher risk of developing osteoporosis.

Calcium is also a key mineral for keeping a regular heartbeat, the healthy clotting of our blood, the contraction of all muscles in the body, the strength of our teeth, as well as for the way our brain chemicals are released.

Because of the fundamental relationship calcium has with a well-functioning heart, the body works very hard to ensure that there is enough circulating in the system to be used. If it detects that there is a deficiency in supply, it will turn to the bones to correct the levels (over 99 per cent of calcium is there), robbing from the bones to feed the cardiovascular system. Calcium also serves as a protectant against high blood pressure and studies have shown its beneficial role in the reduced risk of colon cancer too. So, in short, calcium is vital at this life stage!

Although calcium is the mineral needed in the highest quantity, health is far from all about calcium. Rather calcium cannot do its job without the help of other nutrients, especially when it comes to the process of bone formation. These include magnesium, phosphorus, vitamin D and potassium, as well as manganese, copper, boron, iron, zinc, vitamin A, vitamin K, vitamin C and the B vitamins. Therefore,

I always recommend taking calcium as part of a multi-nutrient or a formulation specifically designed with these nutrients to support bone health, alongside the foundation of a strong, wholesome diet (see food sources below).

Milk, cheese and yoghurt are often thought of as the richest sources of calcium, but other sources include fish with edible bones (such as anchovies, salmon and sardines), green leafy vegetables like kale (ounce for ounce, kale is richer in calcium than milk products). Soy beans, sesame seeds (and tahini paste) are excellent sources too. The additional benefit of these plant-based sources is that they also contain other minerals, including zinc, magnesium, vitamin K, vitamin A, vitamin C, vitamin B12 and phosphorous.

Phytates found in foods such as unleavened wheat in breads, some nuts and seeds, tannins found in tea and coffee, and oxalates found in raw spinach, cauliflower and rhubarb can bind to calcium and other minerals, leaving less for the body to use. To reduce this, avoid drinking tea and coffee within 30 minutes of eating and taking supplements, soak nuts and seeds for around 2 hours prior to consumption to reduce the phytate content and cook oxalate-rich foods.

CALCIUM SUPPLEMENTS

Calcium is readily prescribed to and taken by men and women (especially post-menopausal women) at this stage of life. However, as with all nutrients, there is a vast difference between the calcium you find in food and that in synthetic supplements – the latter being much harder for the body to absorb and use. This can lead to a build-up of calcium and some studies have shown that this can have a detrimental effect on health.

Calcium deposits can also find themselves in the pineal gland responsible for producing melatonin, which may disrupt sleep patterns.

When you get calcium through your diet, you're taking it in small amounts spread throughout the day, along with other food sources and nutrients, which helps you absorb the nutrient. However, supplementation with synthetic calcium is often at a high dose, without the necessary nutrients to suport absorption, including vitamin K and magnesium. Most people can get most of their calcium supply through their diet by consciously building calcium-rich foods into their daily regime. Supplements can be beneficial in building on this foundation, but the source of calcium you take is key here.

High doses (above 1,200mg) of calcium can inhibit the absorption of zinc, so this is another reason to stay away from high dose synthetic forms of calcium. In my opinion, natural forms of calcium extracted from food sources are significantly better for your bones and overall wellbeing.

Most people can achieve the NRV of calcium for adults over 51 years old through a conscious diet and a supplement containing around 150mg of natural sourced calcium.

B vitamins: B vitamins have a range of important functions in the body, including contributing to healthy red blood cells, releasing energy from the foods we eat, normal nerve function and vision, healthy skin, cognitive wellbeing and reducing tiredness. B12 specially provides the myelin sheaths that protect our nerves in the brain and spinal cord from damage. However, studies have shown that many of us are deficient in vitamin B12.

One reason for this widespread deficiency at this stage of life is that many of us lose a protein called intrinsic factor when we age, which transports vitamin B12 from the intestines into the bloodstream. Natural, Food-Grown® supplement forms of vitamin B12 provide more useable forms of B12.

Food sources include:

* **Folate/folic acid:** some green vegetables – like broccoli, cabbage, spring greens and peas – and fortified grains

* **Vitamin B6:** wheatgerm, oatmeal and wholegrain rice, eggs, poultry, fish, soybeans and milk

* **Vitamin B12:** fish, such as sardines and tuna, clams, beef, liver and kidney, eggs, dairy, fortified breakfast cereals and other fortified foods, such as soya drink

Your daily multi-nutrient will provide B vitamins, but there are some circumstances in which extra B vitamins are recommended, such as when following a vegan or vegetarian diet or during times of stress.

MEDICATION

Protein pump inhibitors are a group of medicines used to treat conditions such as reflux, by reducing the production of acidity in the stomach. However, this mechanism also reduces the absorption of vitamin B12 and minerals such as zinc and magnesium from food. Several studies have shown that statin medication reduces the tissue stores of Coenzyme Q10, a key compound used by the body for muscle contractions and energy production, and that taking additional Coenzyme Q10 can reduce the side effects of taking statins, such as muscle weakness, fatigue and inflammation.

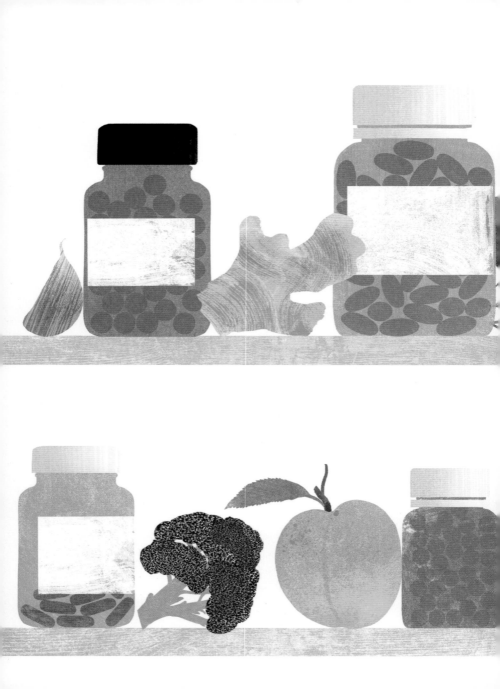

PART THREE

Supplements for Common Complaints

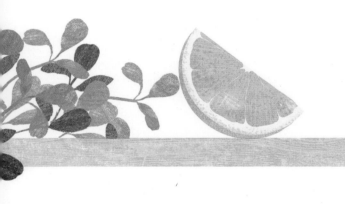

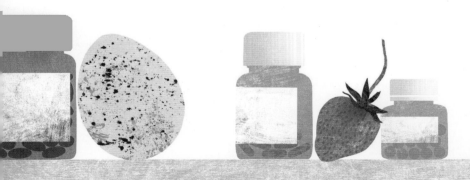

INTRODUCTION

I n this section I will discuss the health issues I am asked about most often, where supplementation with natural, Food-Grown® vitamins and minerals can be very beneficial.

I know that starting to take supplements can feel daunting. The key here is to go slowly and begin simply. Don't be tempted to think more means more; the body is too sophisticated for this and often it needs a mere tweak to return to balance. It will simply eliminate what it doesn't need – a waste of money and, on behalf of your body, a waste of effort to process things it doesn't want. It is far better to invest in one or two good-quality supplements, rather than a raft of synthetic ones that may have limited bioavailability. This way you can sense what is working for your body and what isn't and, if you want to, build from there.

What our bodies do need, however, is for us to be consistent and committed. With consistent supplementation, you can usually expect to begin seeing results in six to eight weeks. You may wish to keep a diary in note form to track your symptoms and any flare-ups, alongside the presence of other things you know to be a factor. Take supplements at a time of the day that you are most likely to remember. For many, this is at breakfast (but take at least 30 minutes away from tea or coffee). Keep them out of direct sunlight and away from heat but do try to find somewhere that is in eye view, which will help you to remember them. I keep mine on the shelf by the mugs in my kitchen, with magnesium, which I take for a good night's sleep, next to my bed. Think about your routines – what can you use as a reminder to ensure you are taking supplements consistently?

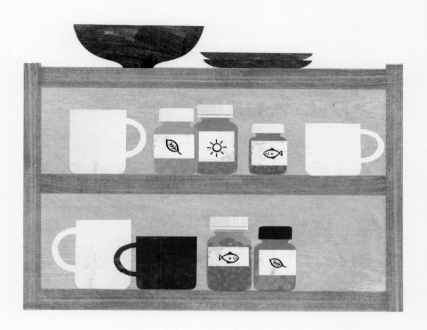

As I have been saying throughout, however, good health is not simply about supplementing our diet – as supportive as it may be. This section of the book focuses on the foundational principles of a healthy diet set out in Part One (see pages 29–43) which are of particular importance when managing a specific health concern. It is worth revisiting these principles often, as they really are the foundation on which all else rests.

Whatever health area you would like to address, it is important to always appreciate and respect how interconnected our bodies' systems are. Hormonal issues may be driving tiredness or skin conditions; osteoporosis may also be connected to digestive health; the brain–gut axis is a powerful but often overlooked connection. Therefore I have made recommendations not just on nutrition and supplements, but also on lifestyle factors, such as breathwork, stress management and sleep.

There are many, many supplements on the market and I know how confusing this can be. Rather than overloading you with information, I have focused on the ones that I have seen to be the most effective. You will see that I always recommend a multi-nutrient and usually omega 3 as a starting point. Look for a multi-nutrient that is formulated to support someone in your time of life. If a product seems to be all bells and whistles, or makes a long list of claims, it may well be too good to be true. I always recommend straightforward, good-quality, natural supplements over highly processed synthetic but heavily marketed products.

If you feel you need further support, or personalised advice specific to you own health issue, it might well be helpful to work with a nutritional therapist or naturopath. Some health brands, including my own Wild Nutrition, offer phone or online support to help you make the right choices. For some health issues, I have suggested tests to provide more information on what the body is not receiving in sufficient amounts or to identify an area of intolerance or imbalance. For example, a food intolerance test for digestive health or a hormonal panel for hormonal challenges. There seems to have been an explosion of tests you can order online now. However, they can be expensive and you want to make sure that it is right for you and of good quality. This is another area in which I advise seeking the support of a nutritional therapist or naturopath, who will be able to help ensure you find out what you want to know.

SKIN HEALTH

The skin is our largest organ and so often it can provide a window to what is going on inside us, physically, emotionally and mentally. Imbalances that we may not know are occurring often make themselves known in this way, so although it can be unpleasant and even upsetting for some to suffer skin complaints, they provide an opportunity and a reminder to look more closely at our overall health and nutritional balance.

It might not be the first thing we think of, but recent research is increasingly outlining a connection between the gut, brain and skin (known as the brain–gut–skin axis). It suggests that stress impacts the amount and diversity of beneficial bacteria in our gut, as well as the permeability of the clever and selective gut membrane, which serves as an interface between inflammatory chemicals produced in the gut and the rest of the body. When we are lacking beneficial bacteria or the gut membrane is compromised, inflammation in the body can result, which may often show itself in skin complaints.

Good skin hygiene is important but it is not often the sole solution and we must be careful of going too far and stripping skin of its natural oils and thereby its means of protection and repair. Topical products containing natural ingredients such as herbs and beneficial bacteria are often best. When antibiotic medication is prescribed, this too can impact the health of beneficial bacteria in the gut, so paying special attention to this when on a course of antibiotics is always recommended.

Skin, as with hair, is often an indicator of wellbeing. Skin and hair follicle cells are usually generated at rapid speed, but this requires a constant supply of nutrients and is seen as a periphery need by the body. So, if the necessary nutrients are in short supply, it is often the skin and hair that suffer, while resources are diverted to other more essential functions, such as the production of bone marrow. This can be why during times of stress, when nutrient demand is high, the quality of our hair, skin or nails can be affected.

So, as with all conditions, healing from skin conditions is both an inside and outside job. I hope the information in this section offers you support for both.

Acne

There are two types of acne: acne rosacea and acne vulgaris. Acne rosacea is mainly superficial and found on the face, where many of the sebaceous glands are, whereas acne vulgaris is more widespread, chronic and affects the chest and back as well as the face and neck.

Causes for both forms can be many and unclear, but it is often down to hormonal changes and usually begins in puberty, although it can also develop in adulthood and later stages of hormonal change, such as perimenopause. These hormonal shifts can increase the secretion of the sebaceous glands, creating blocked pores and, in the case of acne vulgaris, infections. For girls and women, there is a link between acne, overproduction of testosterone and a hormonal condition called polycystic ovary syndrome (see pages 170–72 for more on this).

Some dietary and lifestyle factors can also contribute, including smoking, exposure to pollutants such as dioxins, dairy or a diet high in sugar or carbohydrates. It may also be triggered by stress. Food allergies or sensitivities can cause or aggravate skin conditions, so for some people this is worth exploring.

Eczema

Also known as atopic dermatitis, eczema causes inflammation on the skin, dryness and itching. It's particularly common in infants but can occur at any stage of life. If eczema becomes advanced, the bacteria staphylococcus aureus can develop and colonise on the skin surface, causing the area to be raised, weeping and sore. This increases inflammation and can be resistant to steroid treatment.

Staphylococcus aureus is thought to thrive in skin cells that are low in fatty acids and therefore easier for the bacteria to adhere to. This could be why a deficiency in essential fatty acids (EFAs) seems to contribute to the development of eczema and why, therefore, increasing EFAs through supplementation and diet can be so beneficial.

As previously discussed, skin conditions are so often a reflection of what is happening in the gut. Studies have found a link between compromised digestion and eczema, while more recent research has shown that modulating the balance of bacteria in the gut through changes in diet and supplementation with probiotics and prebiotics (see pages 125–27) can have a positive effect, which is likely due to the immune system's control of inflammation via the gut (Rusu et al., 2019). Food allergies are a common trigger too and this is worth exploring with a nutritional therapist if the lifestyle and diet changes below don't make any difference.

Psoriasis

Psoriasis is an inflammatory disease where new skin cells are produced at a rate around ten times faster than normal. This causes a build-up of skin cells on the skin surface and results in the formation of raised red patches covered with dead cells. It can affect the nails too, pitting and thickening the nails, as well as a form of arthritis known as psoriatic arthropathy.

Psoriasis has been linked with abnormalities in the processing of essential fatty acids. Omega 3 fatty acids (such as EPA and DHA in oily fish) have been shown to dampen down the inflammation associated with psoriasis and decrease the associated itching.

Studies have found a link between compromised digestion and psoriasis, and research has shown benefits from using diet and supplementation with probiotics and prebiotics to positively affect the balance of bacteria in the gut, as the gut plays a big part in the immune system, which controls inflammation. As a result of poor digestive health and leaky gut (see pages 123–24 for more on this), sufferers commonly experience food sensitivities to foods that are high in saturated fats, red and processed meats, dairy products (including cheese), eggs, gluten and refined sugars. Avoiding these foods for a period of time may be necessary to rebalance digestive function and moderate the immune system.

We also know that the skin houses its own immune system via bacteria that populates the skin. In the past, it was thought that the best route to a clean and healthy skin was to sanitise it. However, increasingly, the science is showing us that what we need to do is quite the opposite and topical treatments should support the beneficial bacteria that reside on the skin to control inflammation. Although they often provide temporary and quick relief to surface symptoms such as itching, many topical medications can override this natural immunity and so I recommend using them sparingly while also adopting dietary and lifestyle interventions here. Consider using body products with natural ingredients too.

Lifestyle and diet to support skin health

To address skin concerns and to nourish our skin from the inside out, these are the fundamentals to bear in mind.

* Reduce refined or processed foods. They tend to be lower in quality protein and nutrients such as B vitamins, chromium or magnesium, but they also affect the balance of bacteria in the gut, which can both contribute to and exacerbate symptoms.

* Exposing the skin to sunshine for 15 minutes a day safely, and before the midday sun where possible, will improve vitamin D levels and has been shown to benefit to skin conditions.

* As there is a link between many skin conditions and stress, it may be helpful to build relaxation techniques into your everyday life, such as breathwork exercises or simply taking a walk in a natural environment.

* Regular exercise will encourage the lymphatic system's clearance of waste products. Washing afterwards with natural antibacterial agents such as lavender can also be helpful. Natural washes and shampoos containing calendula or silica can be calming and healing for irritated skin or scalp.

* Drinking five to six glasses of water per day, cold or warm, will promote the clearance of waste products through the liver and kidneys. Celery juices contain psoralen, a compound that has been shown to be especially beneficial in the treatment of psoriasis.

* Build in foods rich in fibre and the minerals zinc and selenium, such as green vegetables, pumpkin, sunflower and sesame seeds and wholegrains. Zinc deficiency has been associated with increased susceptibility to acne but also hormonal imbalances, which may also be at the root of skin issues.

* Increase your intake of foods rich in natural carotenes, found in vegetables coloured yellow, orange and red, as well as green, leafy vegetables – carrots, spinach, lettuce, tomatoes, sweet potatoes, broccoli and winter squash. A key member of the carotenoid family, beta-carotene is converted into vitamin A. Vitamin A deficiency has been associated with a greater susceptibility to acne. These foods also contain vitamin C, which helps to form collagen and improve skin elasticity and connective tissue for scar healing.

* Eat more foods that feed the growth of helpful bacteria in the gut as well as improve gut motility and the removal of waste from the gut. These foods are known as prebiotics. Good

sources are fermented foods such as sauerkraut or kimchi, as well as chicory, artichokes, garlic, oats, leeks, apples and pears.

* Healthy fats from nuts, seeds and oily fish provide essential fats to reduce inflammation and encourage tissue healing.

* Eat a source of protein with every meal. This is an important source of amino acids for building collagen needed to support skin repair. If you are vegan or vegetarian, consider taking a vegan protein powder that includes lysine, an amino acid that is not as available in vegan dietary sources.

Supplements

Natural multi-nutrient for your age stage that contains natural vitamin E and beta-carotene.

Natural zinc – 10mg. Zinc supplementation has been shown to be as effective as oral antibiotics for acne.

Omega 3 fatty acids – 1g per day.

Broad-spectrum probiotic to include lactobacillus and bifidobacterium strains. Take for three months, assess your symptoms and if improvement is still needed, start another three month course. Continue in this way. For eczema especially.

Evening primrose oil – 3g for three months. This contains GLA which can moisturise the skin from the inside out, important for the formation of healthy skin cell membranes, and which reduces itching and dryness in those with EFA deficiency.

Testing

Iron deficiency and thyroid conditions can be at the root
of hair loss and some skin conditions. Food allergies and
sensitivities may also be causing and exacerbating symptoms
(dairy is a common one). There are plenty of tests available,
some of which are more comprehensive and accurate than
others. I recommend exploring this with the support of a
nutritional therapist or naturopath.

A HEALTHY MIND

In the last ten years, there has been a significant amount of
research to determine the link between mind and body, and
it is now clear that there is no divide. We now know for sure
that our physical health affects our mental health and our mental
health affects our physical wellbeing. We will all have witnessed
this interconnectedness during inevitable periods of stress, for
example – not only does our appetite change, our sleep patterns are
disrupted and our mood can change, but we may also experience
digestive changes, heart palpitations or headaches.

We are one mind-body and our thoughts and emotions are not
contained in our head, they are experienced throughout our body.
Nutritional medicine has made substantial progress in exploring the
link between mental and physical health and specifically the role
that diet and lifestyle can play in supporting our mental wellbeing.

When we don't eat enough nutrient-rich food, it affects our
energy, mood and brain function. This is because we may not be
getting the right nutrients and components that we need to make
the brain chemicals which make us feel good, such as serotonin, a
messenger chemical in the brain which improves mood. Serotonin

is made from tryptophan, which we get from the protein in our diet. If we are eating erratically or diets high in processed foods, stimulants and sugar, we may also be ingesting chemicals that interfere with our brain chemistry, as well as causing our bodies to produce stress hormones which can make our mood feel less stable.

So, with all this in mind, balancing the wellbeing of our mind is about balancing the whole body, inside and out, caring for the internal workings with good food and supplementation but also the environment and lifestyle choices that we make each day through the way we move, sleep and think. I hope that the advice in the following pages will give you helpful tips to balance all of these so that you can support your brilliant mind.

Stress and anxiety

Stress and anxiety are not simply in the mind or in the body, they are whole body experiences and can affect every system. For some, symptoms of stress are invisible but for others, it can start to look more like health niggles, such as skin issues, change to digestion, low energy, trouble sleeping, difficulties regulating mood and, in women, changes to how we menstruate.

Importantly, stress also speeds up the body's use and therefore demand for magnesium, vitamin B5 and calcium. It also reduces how efficiently we generate white blood cells (our first line of defence against infection). The production of white blood cells is influenced by our zinc intake, so adding in zinc-rich foods and supplementation can also be helpful. If the body isn't receiving what it needs from food or through supplementation it will start to pull stores from our body tissues; in the long term, this can result in chronic deficiency of important minerals such as calcium and an increased risk of osteoporosis. Stress may also reduce our production of stomach acid and enzymes made within the digestive system needed to break down our food.

According to the 2018 Mental Health Foundation survey, 74 per cent of UK citizens experienced a level of stress in the past year which left them feeling overwhelmed or unable to cope. This extreme stress manifested as anxiety and depression, affecting eating habits and causing an increase in drinking and smoking. Alarmingly, 49 per cent of 18–24-year-olds felt that comparing themselves to others via social media was a substantial source of stress, higher than in any of the older age groups.

There are times in life when stress is unavoidable. However, sometimes being stressed becomes a default mode of thinking and behaving. Busyness and stress can be addictive. So, the first thing to do is to identify the main sources of stress in your life, or things that have a negative effect on how you feel, and then explore ways to help you change their impact as much as you can, or ways to feel more supported to do so.

If you are trying to recover and rebalance your energy, then sleep and rest are the priority, so be mindful of not overfilling your life with activities and social outings. Be selective about when you go out and most evenings after work, go home, eat, relax and go to bed! And most of all, try not to feel guilty about that. For some of us, this can be the hardest one to implement. We are living in an era where 'doing' is valued more than 'being' and this is having a detrimental effect on our mental and physical health. Finding time to rest and simply 'be' will bring about more productivity in the long run. Set aside regular time to do something that you love and that makes you feel good, or try to find a hobby, and don't feel guilty for spending time on yourself. Laughter is highly stress-relieving. Surround yourself with the people that make you smile.

Eating to support most areas of health involves eating only – or mainly – whole, unrefined, unprocessed foods that are nutrient-rich. This is no different for the systems in our bodies which manage stress, called the endocrine system, (specifically the adrenal glands that manage our fight-or-flight hormones) and our nervous system. They need plenty of protein, essential fats, slow-releasing carbohydrates, vitamins, minerals and antioxidants to remain in full health, and especially when they are fatigued or being over-stimulated.

Low mood and depression

Our mood can be affected by many things – hormones, stress, sleep, life worries and experiences such as grief or divorce. A change of mood can happen for us all, but a low mood over an extended period of time may mean that you are experiencing mild depression.

Sometimes it's hard to pinpoint what it is that is making us feel down. Many people have periods of depression in their life. In fact, I would go as far as to say that it is quite normal. We are fearful of low mood in the West because we associate it with something being wrong, but in some cultures these periods are seen as times of needed reflection and an enforced slowing down, a sign that there is something that needs to be processed or felt through. Our lives are often so busy that we may not give ourselves the time that we need to process everything that we feel. These episodes are not always comfortable and need nurturing and support, from those around us but also ourselves. Quiet restorative time is a far cry from laziness. In fact, plotting rejuvenation into your weekly diary is beneficial overall because people tend to make better decisions with a clearer, calmer head.

Some of the signs of depression are below and you will see that they share similarities to stress or exhaustion, both of which can also impact mood, and may be the root cause in some cases:

* Crying and a feeling of inexplicable sadness

* Tiredness and general apathy

* Agitation

* Nervousness and anxiety

* Headaches

* Difficulty concentrating

* Loss of self-esteem and lack of confidence

* Change to libido

* Loss of interest in activities you used to enjoy

* Change to sleep patterns

* Change to appetite

Seasonal affective disorder (SAD) is a form of depression brought on by a change of season into one where there is less light. This is in part because we have less sunlight to stimulate the production of vitamin D and the brain chemical serotonin. The autumn and winter months, when the days are shorter, were traditionally the slower and more reflective times of the year. However, these days, the pace of life rarely abates, leaving very little time for rest and reflection.

Researchers have identified that consistently raised levels of inflammation in the body can cause a lack of energy, sleep disturbances, changes in mood and depressive episodes. Following a nutritional programme tailored to you, that includes an anti-inflammatory and gut-supporting dietary and supplement protocol, can be very supportive.

Tiredness and fatigue

With our busy modern lives, 'feeling tired' can be commonplace and although occasional tiredness is part of living (usually explained by a poor night's sleep or a bout of excess demand, such as exercise), tiredness on a regular, almost daily basis for an extended period is a sign that your body is finding it hard to keep up with demand.

This may be linked to stress, overwork, mild depression and a lack of exercise, as well as a poor diet and linked nutritional deficiencies. However, for some there may also be a medical cause at the root of the tiredness, such as an underactive thyroid, illness or an immune condition, as examples, and so if it is persistent, I always recommend seeking advice from your doctor.

It might seem almost too simple, but feeling tired can be exacerbated or even partly caused by poor hydration. Mild dehydration can reduce energy and focus by 30 per cent. We are often unaware that we are mildly hydrated (by the time we are thirsty we are on the next stage of dehydration), not least because we use more water when we are busy and lifestyle factors such as exercise, drinking caffeine and alcohol can increase this need ever more.

For energy production, we rely on the efficiency of our mitochondria powerhouses (think of them as factory sites for energy production) in each of our cells, which play a fundamental role in optimising available energy as we go about our day. Certain nutrients and enzymes play a huge role in mitochondrial health, and so looking at the food we eat is a very good place to start.

The key nutrients directly required for energy production are vitamin B12, magnesium and iron, but a raft of other nutrients support this process, including vitamin D, calcium and the rest of the B vitamin family, such as vitamin B5. A diet of lean protein, fresh vegetables and unrefined complex carbohydrates such as wholegrains or wholewheat will be rich in the nutrients and amino acids needed to support healthy energy levels.

Difficulty sleeping

Many people will experience a time in their life when their sleep is disrupted – I remember all too clearly how sleep becomes the holy grail as a new parent. It is a foundation of daily wellbeing and research has shown that when we don't get enough of it, of the right quality and at the right time, it can affect our mental and physical wellbeing, from cardiovascular disease and diabetes to depression and fertility.

Unfortunately, certain life stages, such as puberty, pregnancy and perimenopause or menopause, can impact our sleep, as can high stress levels or a change in environment. Seasonal change can also vary our sleep, with reduced exposure to sunlight affecting the production of melatonin.

The hormone melatonin plays a major role in our sleeping and waking cycles and its production is controlled by exposure to light. This means as it starts to get dark in the evening (or we are exposed to less light) melatonin secretion rises to assist us in feeling tired, eventually helping us to fall asleep. Conversely, in the morning when we wake up, exposure to light shuts melatonin production down so that we can stop feeling sleepy and get out of bed.

One of the most common symptoms associated with melatonin deficiency is not feeling sleepy enough to wind down and go to bed. Modern living, diet and low levels of certain nutrients can all influence how well we are able to produce melatonin when we need it. Even if you do not have issues around sleep, melatonin plays other significant roles in the following areas of health:

* The timing and release of female reproductive hormones – particularly ovulation

* The rate of internal ageing

* Disease development

* How we experience jetlag

* Low levels are linked to mood disorders and depression

Melatonin is synthesised in the body from another hormone (or neurotransmitter) called serotonin – often best known as the 'happy hormone'. If we go further back along the human biochemical pathway, we require minerals such as iron and B vitamins to turn serotonin into melatonin. Therefore, it's helpful to include these nutrients in your diet as they assist with how you should naturally feel before bed.

The average adult sleeps between six and eight hours per night. In the past, the focus has been on the length of time asleep as an indicator of a 'good night's sleep'; however, more recent theories support quality rather than quantity, with six hours of deep, restorative sleep being preferable to eight lower quality hours. Furthermore, research published in the *Sleep Health Journal* has also shown that the hours of 10.45pm to 6.45am are the optimum times of sleep. Sleep architecture can change with age too, and over the age of 70 we may need only five good-quality hours' sleep. It is thought that over the age of 70, we naturally spend more time in the shallower stages of sleep rather than the deeper sleep stages and therefore it is not uncommon or wrong to wake several times in the night at this age.

The benchmark of whether we have had enough or good enough sleep across any age is whether we feel energised and refreshed the following day. If you regularly have trouble sleeping and rarely feel refreshed after a night's sleep, then you may be experiencing insomnia, which is defined as an extended period of trouble falling asleep, staying asleep or getting good-quality sleep. This is an often complex issue that requires specific, holistic support, and a report by the Mental Health Foundation found that one third of people in the UK will experience it at some point. The recommendations below can help with insomnia, as well as shorter periods of disturbed sleep.

You may have heard the common sleep advice that the hours you are asleep before midnight are worth double those afterwards. This has not been scientifically proven (although many people do feel better opting for this routine) but what is scientifically understood is that the first third of our sleep is the most restorative. To best support this 'first third', experts recommend reducing presleep stress as much as we can. In addition, keep to a regular sleep/ wake cycle, even at the weekends. This has been shown to get the circadian rhythms into a more predictable pattern.

Cut out the blue light before bed
Light of any kind affects the rise of melatonin, but research shows that blue light emitted from the screens of devices such as computers, laptops, smartphones, tablets and televisions has the most negative impact.

You can protect yourself from blue light by either avoiding those devices (which is not always possible) or by wearing special glasses when looking at them. These can be purchased online and look like regular sunglasses but will be labelled as 'blue light blocking'. I recommend wearing them from around 6 or 7pm for any duration of screen use, even if it's five minutes on your phone. Research has shown that blue light exposure 45 minutes before going to bed can reduce your production of melatonin by up to 82 per cent and impact your food choices the following day (Wahl et al., 2019).

Increase your exposure to natural light
As far as is possible, it's worth trying to mimic the way we used to live before we had access to modern electrical light. When electrical lighting didn't exist (or was not as bright) people would have gone to bed earlier and risen earlier to make the most of natural daylight. These days, we push our waking hours late into the night because there is no limit to the amount of light available. If you are experiencing sleeping issues, sleep experts suggest trying to change your body clock to fit better with natural circadian rhythms of rising with the light and going to bed earlier – including at weekends (no lie-in!). This can be hard for the first week, but after a while, your body clock will come around.

It's worth investing in blackout blinds to keep all streetlight out of your bedroom and, as soon as your alarm goes off in the morning, opening the curtains to allow light to flood in to suppress melatonin production to help you wake up. During the darker winter months, some people invest in special lamps that mimic dawn light and progression to daylight, which can be effective for many. Increasing your exposure to natural light during the day has been shown to improve sleep by 80 per cent and two hours in some studies (Blume et al., 2019).

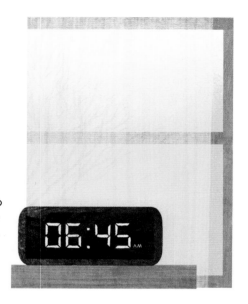

Meditation or a practice of stillness or mindfulness
Bringing your awareness inward while meditating allows you to feel any unprocessed feelings stored in the body, better preparing your mind and body for rest. Staying with your feelings with total loving awareness allows emotions to rise, digest and fall away.

Don't use sleep as your only method to rest
Sleep and rest are important and different activities. Be selective about when you go out and most evenings after work go home, eat, relax and go to bed early to get eight hours' sleep. Avoid checking emails or making plans late into the evening. Find ways that work for you to switch off from the stresses of the day as much as possible, such as listening to music or taking a hot bath with essential oils or magnesium salts. Gentle movement such as some stretching or yoga can help to ease any tension from the day.

Balance your blood sugar
And don't eat a heavy meal less than three hours before bed. Blood sugar highs and lows can affect sleep and cause waking in the early hours. Eat meals that are balanced with lean protein and wholegrains, avoiding sugar and alcohol.

Look at your caffeine intake
Caffeine stimulates your nervous system and may stop your body from naturally relaxing at night. Caffeine levels can stay elevated in your blood for six to eight hours after consumption, so if you are having problems sleeping, avoid caffeine from lunchtime.

Cat nap
Short power naps – less than 30 minutes – have been shown to be beneficial for quality sleep. However, be mindful not to sleep too long or too close to your normal bedtime because this has been shown to negatively affect night-time sleep. A typical post-lunch siesta appears to be the most popular.

Spring-clean your sleeping environment
Consider your sleeping environment and anything you might try to make it a calming place of restoration. Minimise external noise, light and artificial lights from devices like alarm clocks. Consider your bedding and your pillows too, and whether it may be time for an update to improve your comfort.

Memory

Poor memory is a common complaint, particularly due to tiredness and stress. It can become more noticeable as we age and be affected by hormone changes. Genetics may also play a role, especially in more serious neurological conditions such as Alzheimer's, but increasingly research is showing that diet and lifestyle can also have a significantly positive impact. (Just to be clear, I am addressing the more lightweight issues of memory here, but there is much that can be done through dietary and lifestyle intervention for those experiencing more neurological conditions too. I highly recommend working with a nutritional therapist, naturopath or Functional Medicine practitioner to see how this may support you.)

Changes to blood sugar, through erratic eating or missed meals, nutrient deficiencies and poor hydration can also affect our memory.

Deficiencies in vitamins such as vitamin B1 and 5, as well as essential fatty acids which power the transport of hormones and brain chemicals responsible for memory, can be part of the trouble and it is well worth addressing these factors as a starting point. Vitamin D deficiency too has been linked to memory and so adopting the lifestyle recommendations to spend time outdoors as well as increasing your intake of protein and vitamin D-rich foods can be helpful.

Lifestyle and diet to support mood, energy and sleep

▽ Diet

Here is a reminder of the key points from the foundations of a healthy diet set out in Part One which are of particular importance when it comes to improving energy and reducing tiredness:

Foods rich in B vitamins
B vitamins are essential for energy production and the normal functioning of the nervous system – vitamin B5 in particular. Good sources include wholegrains, eggs, beans and

lentils, a wide range of vegetables, fish and meats. Taking a B vitamin complex can be very supportive.

Magnesium-rich foods
Magnesium is essential for energy production and for our adrenal hormones and is quickly used up when we are stressed. The best examples are nuts and seeds (especially pumpkin seeds and hemp seeds, such as in the form of hemp protein powder), buckwheat groats or flour (buckwheat is a seed and not related to wheat), greens such as spinach and kale, and fish and seafood.

Vitamin C-rich foods
Another nutrient that is vital for the manufacture of adrenal hormones. Fruits and vegetables are the best source but contrary to popular belief, oranges do not have the highest levels. Better sources include peppers, kale, broccoli, Brussels sprouts, watercress and red cabbage. Go easy on the fruit, as it can be high in sugar – no more than two pieces per day is best for most people.

Healthy fats
Healthy fats from nuts, seeds and oily fish provide essential fats to support our mood and brain health. This is well documented in research, but I have seen this evidenced with the women and men I have worked with too. Aim for a source of healthy fats in at least one meal per day.

Lean proteins
Quality proteins provide the building blocks of our brain chemicals. Lean proteins like fish and chicken provide a complete mix of amino acids, zinc and iron required for the building blocks of neurotransmitters, including serotonin and dopamine. Eggs are also rich in zinc, iron, vitamin D and vitamin B12, as well as tryptophan to boost serotonin levels. Quinoa is rich in protein and minerals such as magnesium and B vitamins needed to

produce anti-anxiety brain chemicals, including GABA. Use as an alternative to rice or wheat pasta for managing anxiety and stress. If you are vegan or vegetarian, consider taking a vegan protein powder that includes lysine, an amino acid which is less available in vegan dietary sources.

Look after your gut

Have you ever wondered why it is often our digestive system that reacts to how we feel? For example, if we are nervous or anxious, we may experience butterflies in the stomach or a change to our bowel function such as diarrhoea or constipation. This is because a significant part of our nervous system resides in our gut, so much so that researchers are now calling the gut the 'second brain'. The gut is where over 95 per cent of serotonin is synthesised, the brain chemical that impacts our mood if it is too low or too high. There is also a direct communication line between the gut and the brain called the vagus nerve.

As a result, there is a lot of scientific interest in the links between mood and the gut microbiome (the trillions of bacteria resident in the human colon) and studies on probiotics have shown improvement in anxiety, mood and stress. Low levels of beneficial bacteria in the gut have been associated with an increased addiction to stimulants. Meta-analysis showed that probiotic intake reduced psychological symptoms of depression, anxiety and perception of stress (Jafari, A. et al., 2022). Eat more foods that feed the growth of helpful bacteria in the gut, including fermented foods such as sauerkraut or kimchi, as well as chicory, artichokes, garlic, oats, leeks, apples and pears.

Stress and anxiety must be tackled holistically, but paying attention to a few key areas and avoiding living in 'stress mode' as a default, with our fight, flight or freeze mechanism always activated.

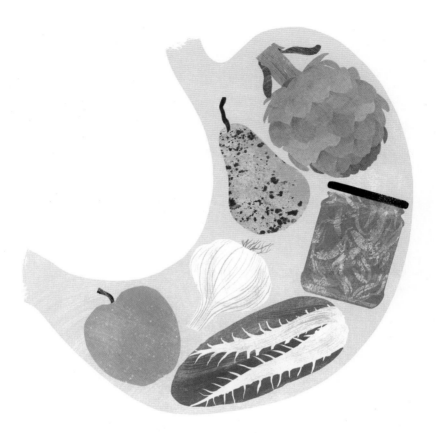

Sleep

Melatonin is an antioxidant and influences hormones that regulate anxiety and fear. Aim to be in bed by 11pm at the latest, even if you tend to feel more energetic at this time than at other times of the day; staying up past midnight or burning the candle at both ends is a disaster for our adrenal health. Turn off any computers or tablets, and preferably the television, at least two hours before going to bed. The bright light that they emit can block the production of melatonin, the hormone which regulates the sleep-wake cycle and makes us feel sleepy at night-time. Try using dim lighting later in the evening. It's important to note that when melatonin is suppressed, cortisol rises and for women, this can interfere with progesterone and, long term, our hormonal balance.

Get regular exercise

Just like a healthy diet, exercise is vital for many aspects of our health. It can lower levels of stress hormones such as cortisol, help to relax tight muscles and increase our levels of endorphins – chemicals that give us a sense of wellbeing. Walking, swimming, a gentle jog, a dance class, or some form of yoga can be excellent types of exercise to relieve stress. Exercising outside can be very grounding and studies have shown that being exposed to a green environment on a regular basis can help us to adjust our perception of stress to something less threatening. A minimum of 10–15 minutes a day can increase resistance to stress, but 30 minutes is ideal and has been shown to significantly improve mood and our perception of stress. This can also be walking, gardening or exercising outside.

It can be best to avoid more vigorous exercise such as spinning, fast running or squash if you are going through a very stressful time or suffer from adrenal fatigue, as these types of activities tend to further stimulate the adrenal glands. Meditation, deep breathing, yoga, listening to relaxing music, or hypnotherapy recordings designed to help relaxation, may all be able to help. It gives you an opportunity to reflect and evaluate whether what you perceive to be a threat – emotional, physical, spiritual – is in fact something you can address and change, or indeed, if it is a real threat at all.

Focus on creating mental ease

Protect your energy and me time by putting simple boundaries in place. For example, aim for nights of the week where you have a complete break from social media or phone conversations. Instead, have a bath, practise some yoga/stretching and make a nourishing meal. This will also support a good sleep routine. If evenings are often about overstimulation, this will have a negative effect on the part of the nervous system that supports our rest and digestion. It's vital to respect the need for not just sleep itself, but the hours before. See page 109 for more.

Find structure in your day and something to be grateful for. Having a regular routine – for example around exercise – can help to develop a positive and optimistic mindset, while keeping a gratitude list can help us see the cracks of light. It's very easy to say all the things about ourselves or our life that we don't like or wish were better; instead, what about also making a point of thinking of three things you do like and feel grateful for?

Supplements

Natural multi-nutrient – containing 10mcg of vitamin D, iron and zinc. Zinc deficiency has been shown to affect the efficacy of SSRI medication and therefore a multi-nutrient containing 5–10mg of zinc should be considered if you are also taking SSRI antidepressants.

Natural B complex – B vitamins, magnesium and calcium are essential for energy production, for the normal functioning of the nervous system. Vitamin B5 is responsible for generating stress hormones including cortisol, and research has shown there's a link between low folic acid, B12 and low mood.

Natural magnesium – Magnesium is essential for energy production and the production of neurotransmitters, including dopamine and serotonin. It is quickly used up when we are stressed. Take 80mg per day, in the evening, to support a good night's rest.

Omega 3 oils – Benefits have been seen from taking high dose DHA and EPA essential fatty acids (see pages 56–7), as they help good bacteria stick to the gut wall, reduce pro-inflammatory cytokines and improve brain function. I recommend 2g of omega 3 per day, providing at least 1,000mg of EPA and 800mg of DHA.

Ashwagandha – Research has shown it to act in a similar way to the naturally produced amino acid GABA (gamma aminobutyric acid), which works as a chemical messenger to calm the nervous system and help with feelings of stress or anxiety. Ashwagandha has been shown to increase focus and energy. The KSM-66 organic ashwagandha used by Wild Nutrition has had over 11 double-blind, placebo-controlled studies that have demonstrated its ability to reduce anxiety, depression and stress by 71.6 per cent over eight weeks. Aim for 600mg per day.

Medicinal mushrooms – Medicinal mushrooms have traditionally been used for millennia to support many imbalances in the body, from cardiovascular health to supporting the immune and hormonal systems. However, a common use of medicinal mushrooms today is for supporting mood and stress. Reishi is one variety of mushroom that has been well documented for this and one study showed that reishi mushroom reduced symptoms of anxiety and mild depression in four weeks (Matsuzaki, 2013). Doses vary on the type of reishi mushroom and I recommend speaking with a naturopath or nutritional therapist to get the dose that is right for you.

Broad-spectrum probiotic – Probiotics in the form of supplements or food can be helpful in re-inoculating the gut. As more is understood about the complexity of the human microbiome, we are also recognising that strains of beneficial flora work best in synergy. Look for complexes with multiple strains, such as those containing lactobacillus, bifidobacterium and streptococcus strains. Studies have shown improvement with 60billion CFU per day. Take for 3 months, assess your symptoms and continue if you need to.

Additional supplements for low mood and anxiety specifically:

Safr'Inside™ saffron extract – Doses of 30mg per day over six weeks have been shown to be comparable to Fluoxetine and Imipramine, the main pharmaceutical drugs used to treat anxiety and depressive syndromes.

5HTP – 5 hydroxytryptophan is a compound made by the body to build tryptophan and therefore serotonin. It is available to take in supplement form too and doses of 150–300mg a day in total (split into three doses) can be effective within 3 months.

St John's Wort – This has been shown to be effective at treating mild to moderate depression and anxiety. Look for a product that contains around 900mcg of hypericin. It can interfere with some medications, though, so do consult your GP before taking it.

Additional supplements to aid sleep:

Valerian root – 500mg before bed has been shown to improve the speed at which you fall asleep and how long you stay asleep.

L-theanine – can improve relaxation and sleep. Take 100–200mg before bed.

Lavender – A powerful herb with many health benefits, lavender can have a calming and sedentary effect to improve sleep. Take 80–160 mg containing 25–46 per cent linalool, a compound extracted from the plant.

Vitamin D – helps to regulate melatonin and serotonin and deficiency has been associated with poor sleep quality. Make sure it is included in your multi-nutrient or take as an additional supplement. It may be worth checking your vitamin D status with your GP too.

 Testing

See the box on iron deficiency anaemia opposite, as this can be an underlying cause of fatigue. Too much iron is neither necessary nor beneficial and so it is a good idea to know for sure if you need to supplement iron over and above your diet and a multi-nutrient. You may want to consider getting tested for vitamin 12, folate and Vitamin D. These can be tested through your GP surgery or via a private laboratory.

If issues persist you may wish to check for food sensitivities. Gluten sensitivity can not only reduce absorption of nutrients from the diet but also increase the inflammatory process.

IRON DEFICIENCY: ANAEMIA

Red blood cells transport oxygen from your lungs to the different tissues around your body. There, they swap the oxygen for carbon dioxide. Anaemia is when your blood is low in red blood cells (from heavy blood loss, for example). Symptoms such as extreme fatigue are the result of a lack of oxygen as well as a build-up of carbon dioxide.

Iron deficiency anaemia is due to a nutrient deficiency in iron. It is not uncommon to experience iron deficiency anaemia post-birth or if you have heavy menstrual bleeding. A blood test from your doctor will be able to confirm this. If you are found to be deficient in iron, you'll need to take an additional natural iron supplement (see page 59 for information about the different sources of iron), alongside a good multi-nutrient or B complex that contains vitamin B12 and folic acid, which are also needed for healthy red blood cell production.

BODY HEALTH

In orthodox medicine, we often isolate areas of the body or conditions, as though a health issue is confined to one area alone. You might go and see a rheumatologist for an inflammatory condition such as osteoarthritis, for example, but what if your symptoms were being driven by the long period of stress you are experiencing at work, or unaddressed irritable bowel syndrome?

The truth is that not one system in our body works in isolation, and that to support whole health, we need to address the body and mind as a macrocosm, a living, breathing network of systems that all relate to one another. So, when we address joint pain or cholesterol, we must look to see if there are any contributing imbalances elsewhere in the body. We must also explore factors outside of the body, such as how much and well we move, the foods we cook and eat, supplements that we take and our current frame of mind.

Digestion

A properly functioning digestive system is critical to good health. In fact, problems with the gastrointestinal (GI) tract can cause more than just stomach ache or diarrhoea. GI issues may underlie several other chronic health problems that seem unrelated to digestive health, including autoimmune diseases such as rheumatoid arthritis and type 1 diabetes, skin problems such as eczema and acne rosacea, and heart disease (to name just a few).

The gut is also known as the 'second brain' because it has many of the neurotransmitters also found in the brain. This explains the idea of having 'butterflies in your tummy' or a 'gut instinct' and further explains the link between emotions and gut function.

There are a number of causes of digestive imbalance and natural remedies that can support a return to healthy digestive function. However, it is important not to overlook other factors, such as stress. This can either increase motility (the rhythmic flow) of the colon or decrease it, causing constipation, diarrhoea, increased bloating or flatulence – all common symptoms in those with IBS.

Digestive enzymes are the catalyst of food digestion. A lack of digestive enzymes or hydrochloric acid (stomach acid) may also contribute to the poor breakdown of carbohydrates, fats and proteins, causing regular bloating or belching after eating, undigested food in your stools and making you feel easily full. A change to digestive enzyme production and stomach acid levels can be low due to varying factors (age, prescription medication, an over-alkalised diet), resulting in poor protein digestion and digestion in general. Stomach acid also acts as a barrier to harmful bacteria and other microbes, as well as playing a vital role in the utilisation of minerals such as zinc from food. Therefore, low stomach acid may also result in a lower immune tolerance to bacterial and viral infection or in experiencing small intestinal bacterial overgrowth.

IBS

Irritable bowel syndrome (IBS) is a condition that affects the large intestine and colon. According to the charity Guts, over a third of the population claim to be affected by it and over 15 per cent are diagnosed by their doctor. However, it is often used as an umbrella diagnosis to cover a cluster of different symptoms, including chronic change to bowel habits (persisting for over 12 weeks), cramping, bloating and wind. It is regularly diagnosed but rarely investigated to find the root of the cause; instead, anti-spasmodic or other medications are often prescribed for the symptoms. However, it is always a sign of something else going on, such as an imbalance in beneficial bacteria, an overgrowth of less beneficial bacteria, a food sensitivity or stress.

Again, we need to make sure we take into consideration the wider health picture. Those with IBS will know that it is often triggered or exacerbated by stress. Psychotherapy in the form of relaxation therapy, biofeedback, counselling or stress management training has been shown to reduce the symptoms of IBS. Pay attention to lifestyle choices and consider adaptogenic agents such as ashwagandha – see below.

Intestinal permeability or leaky gut syndrome

Intestinal permeability (also colloquially known as leaky gut syndrome) is the underlying cause of many digestive disorders, as well as many other seemingly unrelated conditions from autism to autoimmune conditions. This is when the selectively permeable membrane that lines the wall of your gut becomes less selective and more permeable, allowing particles to travel across the gut wall and into the bloodstream, in the form of either part-digested products or waste that would ordinarily be eliminated through the faeces.

Help the lining of the GI tract to repair itself by supplying key nutrients that can often be in short supply, such as:

* Zinc
* Antioxidants (eg vitamins A, C and E)
* Fish oil

Plus the amino acid glutamine found in lean proteins such as:

* Fish
* Chicken
* Lamb
* Fresh meat stocks and broths

▽ Diet

Follow the foundations of a healthy diet set out in Part One. Here is a reminder of the key points that are of particular importance for digestive health, as well as specific foods that can be helpful.

Beneficial bacteria
Help beneficial bacteria flourish by ingesting probiotic foods or supplements that contain the so-called 'good' GI bacteria, such as bifidobacteria and lactobacillus species, and by consuming the high-

soluble-fibre foods that good bugs like to eat, called prebiotics.

Probiotics are beneficial microorganisms found in the gut, which are also called friendly bacteria. It's worth remembering that taking antibiotics kills both good and bad bacteria, so GI issues such as diarrhoea or increased bloating or flatulence can occur as a result of treatment for another health issue for which antibiotics have been prescribed.

Probiotics in the form of supplements or food, such as yoghurt or cheese, can be helpful in re-inoculating the gut. Probiotic powders are versatile and argued by some experts to be more effectively utilised by the body in a free powder or liquid form.

As more is understood about the complexity of the human microbiome, we are also recognising that strains of beneficial flora work best in synergy, so look for complexes with multiple strains, such as those containing lactobacillus, bifidobacterium and streptococcus strains.

Prebiotics
Prebiotics are non-digestible food ingredients that feed beneficial bacteria and therefore the growth and diversity of our microbiome. Prebiotics are available in many foods that contain a fibre called inulin, including garlic, leeks, onions, rocket, chicory and artichokes; in one recent study, artichoke supplements were found to produce an overall reduction in IBS symptoms by 41 per cent within an average of eight weeks (Bundy et al., 2004). Grains such as barley, flax, oats and fermented grains or cereals, such as sourdough bread, are also classed as prebiotics, as are fermented foods including yoghurt, kefir, miso and tempeh. If you do not have these in your diet regularly, add them in slowly to avoid a strong reaction – often in the style of flatulence and bloating! This is not a sign that you should avoid it, more a sign to acclimatise slowly to regular consumption of these foods.

Another good prebiotic source is a supplement called fructo-oligosaccharide or FOS, but use carefully – FOS in supplement form has been shown to encourage the growth of some unwanted bacteria. I recommend building FOS in through the diet alone with the foods above.

Incorporate liberal amounts of the following into your diet:

* Olive oil – contains oleic acid, an anti-fungal agent. Choose cold-pressed extra virgin olive oil.

* Raw garlic – allicin in raw garlic is also a potent anti-fungal.

* Lemon – add lemon zest and juice into food or in hot drinks.

* Apple cider vinegar – drink one capful in warm water or use in dressings as you would lemon juice.

* Green tea – loose leaf green tea (max three cups per day) has anti-microbial properties.

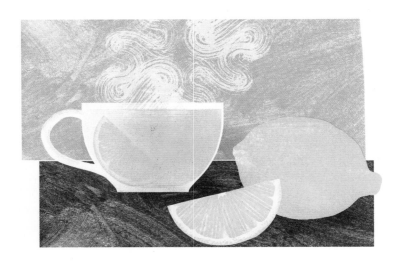

Herbs and spices – Many herbs and spices have natural plant compounds that help to us to break down and absorb the goodness from our food as well as offering calming properties for more inflammatory conditions such as IBD or Crohn's. Of particular benefit are fennel, dill, peppermint, lemon balm, thyme, ginger and cardamom.

Supplements

Aloe vera – Aloe vera is a plant that naturally contains chemicals known as polysaccharides, which can have a soothing and healing effect on mucous membranes, including the surface of the gut wall.

Slippery elm – is categorised as a 'mucilage' and has been found in research to affect the reflux stimulation of nerve endings in the gastrointestinal tract, leading to increased mucus secretion, which is needed to protect the gut wall.

Glutamine – is the most abundant amino acid found in the mucosa (the lining of the gut) and supplementing can be especially helpful for restoring healthy gut permeability. It is easy and safe to use at higher doses (around 5–10g per day).

Digestive enzymes – A full-spectrum digestive enzyme product can be useful here, or if you feel that you would benefit from a specific formulation, I recommend seeking advice from a qualified nutritional therapist or naturopath. Betaine hydrochloride mimics stomach acid and can be taken short term to re-establish stomach acid production.

Testing

There are now quite a few tests that can uncover whether an intolerance to a certain food may be exacerbating your symptoms. There are also stool tests available that can see the health of your gut, your diversity of bacteria and any problematic parasites, yeast or bacteria. However I suggest that you seek the support of a nutritional therapist or naturopath to make these recommendations and support the results with a plan that is specific to you.

Osteoporosis and osteopenia

Bone is a living tissue made up of a network of collagen fibres filled with mineral salts. The most abundant of these is calcium phosphate. These minerals are broken down and replaced on a continual basis. When this balance is lost and not enough bone mineralisation occurs, bone density conditions can develop, including osteoporosis and osteopenia.

Osteoporosis and osteopenia are a thinning of the bones and are largely preventable or manageable through diet and lifestyle. While osteoporosis is the term used when bones have already begun to weaken, osteopenia is the early stages of mineral and protein loss from the bone. Not everyone with osteopenia develops osteoporosis and it can be an opportunity to make some lifestyle and dietary changes to prevent this from happening.

It's important to know that there is a link between hormonal changes and bone density. Women transitioning into and past the menopause can be more vulnerable to thinning bones. Foods naturally rich in phytoestrogens, including chickpeas, tofu and flaxseeds, have been shown to help, as has supplementation with plant isoflavones, as they can mimic the protective action that oestrogen has on bone remineralisation. (See the sections on menopause and perimenopause for more.)

⬭ Diet

Vitamin D
This is essential for the absorption of calcium and phosphate, and to regulate blood levels of calcium and phosphorus (which are needed to build bone). Ensuring you have a good supply of vitamin D from your diet as well as through supplementation is essential and can reduce the risk of hip fracture in older people and even reduce incidences of falling.

Essential fatty acids
Found in oily fish as well as flaxseed oil, essential fatty acids have also been shown to increase calcium deposits in the bone.

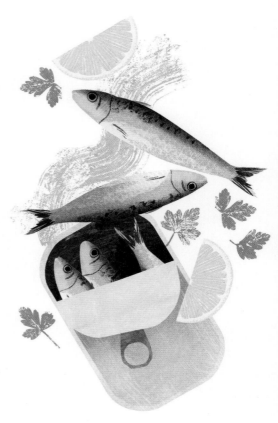

EPA (eicosapentaenoic acid) particularly, which is found in oily fish, can be converted by the body into substances that help to control inflammation. Sources of omega 3 are also good sources of magnesium, zinc and calcium, which are important for bone health. To get more omega 3, eat oily fish two or three times a week.

Protein
In bone, protein makes up a major part of the mass and volume, creating a meshwork of fibres that lay the foundation for growth – think of protein as the scaffolding on which calcium and phosphorous then form bone. Milk, cheese and yoghurt are often considered to be the richest sources of calcium, but other sources include fish with edible bones (such as salmon and sardines), green leafy vegetables like kale (ounce for ounce, kale is richer in calcium than milk products), soybeans and sesame seeds (and tahini paste). The additional benefit of these plant-based sources is that they also contain other minerals, including zinc, magnesium, vitamin K, vitamin A, vitamin C, vitamin B12 and phosphorous.

Other micronutrients are key for bone health too
These include boron, vitamin C, copper, silica, strontium, vitamin K, folic acid, magnesium, manganese and zinc.

Phytates found in foods such as unleavened wheat in breads, some nuts or seeds, tannins in tea and coffee, and oxalates in raw spinach, cauliflower and rhubarb can bind to calcium and other minerals, making them less supportive of bone health. To reduce this, drink tea and coffee at least 30 minutes before or after having food or supplements, soak nuts and seeds to reduce the phytate content and cook oxalate-rich foods.

☀ Lifestyle

Exercise – A combination of regular weight-bearing and muscle-strengthening exercises is important to help build bone density. Exercising outside helps with your vitamin D levels and acts as a good reducer of stress too.

Avoid smoking – Smoking slows down the cells that build bone in your body. This means smoking could reduce your bone strength and increase your risk of breaking a bone, especially if you are nearing menopause.

Reduce alcohol and caffeine – Drinking a lot of alcohol increases your risk of osteoporosis. The government recommends no more than 14 units of alcohol per week. High caffeine intake has been associated with mineral loss, including calcium, so drink caffeine mindfully.

Bring in the rainbow – Vegetables and fruits are high in vitamin C, which is essential for collagen production and the health of cartilage. Each 'colour' within a vegetable provides a different array of natural anti-inflammatory chemicals called phytochemicals, such as flavonoids. Vitamin C and beta-carotene are just some of the antioxidants found in fruit and veg that can be used to build bone. The deeper-growing root vegetables, such as sweet potatoes and squashes, are also excellent sources of trace minerals needed to support bone density (particularly important in cases of osteoarthritis or osteopenia).

Minimise carbonated drinks – These contain phosphoric acid and consuming too much will encourage the leaching of calcium from the bones. This is not an issue if you drink carbonated drinks occasionally, but a daily habit is of more concern.

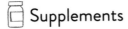 Supplements

Multi-nutrient – containing 10mcg of vitamin D, vitamin B12, vitamin C and vitamin E.

A good-quality bone formulation – including calcium, magnesium, vitamin D, vitamin K, boron, silica, selenium, manganese, copper and zinc. Women should consider an isoflavone formula containing 50–100mg of plant-based isoflavones.

 Testing

You may want to consider assessing your vitamin D levels. This can be done through your GP surgery or through a private laboratory.

Joint pain

Painful, inflamed joints can occur at any stage of life and can be triggered by injury or conditions such as arthritis, fibromyalgia, tendonitis, bursitis or rheumatoid arthritis.

With around 10 million people experiencing symptoms of arthritis in the UK alone, joint health problems are a common complaint in GP surgeries. However, this is not the preserve of the elderly as is often thought. In fact, joint degeneration and indeed autoimmune related joint concerns such as rheumatoid arthritis can begin at any age.

Weight-bearing joints, such as the feet and knees, as well as the hands are the most affected, simply from the degeneration of the tissue and synovial fluid over time. Synovial fluid is the 'oil' that lubricates the joints, while cartilage provides a cushioning effect. When cartilage and synovial fluid begin to degenerate naturally with age, the bones begin to harden and stiffen from lack of lubrication and cushioning. This causes pain and stiffness, which can start subtly and then progress to interfere with movement. This may be exacerbated if you have a lifestyle that has put excessive pressure on these joints.

There is a connection between joint inflammation and the menopause. Oestrogen has a moderating effect on inflammation and therefore, as oestrogen levels change in menopause, inflammation can be less controlled and existing inflammation-based conditions such as arthritis or rheumatoid arthritis can worsen.

Rheumatoid arthritis is an autoimmune disease that affects the entire body, but especially the synovial fluid around the joints. As well as joint pain, it also causes fatigue, fever and weakness. It is thought to be the result of an underactive immune system (and therefore an inability to sweep up inflammatory chemicals) rather than an overactive one. There is also a link between developing RA and a previous infection with the Epstein Barr virus (EBV), indicated in chronic fatigue, ME and glandular fever (in one study, over 80 per cent of RA sufferers showed antibodies to EBV). If you are experiencing RA, I highly recommend consulting a nutritional therapist, as sensitivities to common foods such as gluten or eggs can often exacerbate symptoms.

▽ ☼ Diet and lifestyle

Looking after our joints through diet and lifestyle from a young age is a very powerful preventative measure, as well as effective support for existing conditions.

Reduce stress where possible
Stress can cause an increase in the rate of oxidative damage,
and preliminary research has shown a connection between stress
and autoimmune inflammatory conditions such as psoriatic and
rheumatoid arthritis.

Weight
Maintaining a healthy weight through good nutrition and exercise
will help countless areas of our health. However, if you are
overweight and suffering from osteoarthritis, in particular, weight
loss will help to reduce the strain on your joints.

Eat a variety of fruit and veg
Vegetables and fruits are high in vitamin C, which is essential
for collagen production and the health of cartilage. Each 'colour'
within a vegetable provides a different array of natural anti-
inflammatory chemicals called phytochemicals, such as flavonoids.
They are also rich in a variety of antioxidants (such as vitamin C
or beta-carotene) to quench free radicals that can exacerbate
inflammation and damage to the joints. The deeper-growing
root vegetables such as sweet potatoes or squashes are also an
excellent source of trace minerals needed to support the immune
system and bone density (particularly important in cases of
osteoarthritis or osteopenia).

I recommend aiming for five to seven servings (a dessertspoon
size each) of mixed coloured vegetables per day. Soups or roasted
root vegetables can be an excellent way to achieve this during
the colder months, and if made with fresh meat stock, soups
will have the added benefit of amino acids needed for cartilage
production too.

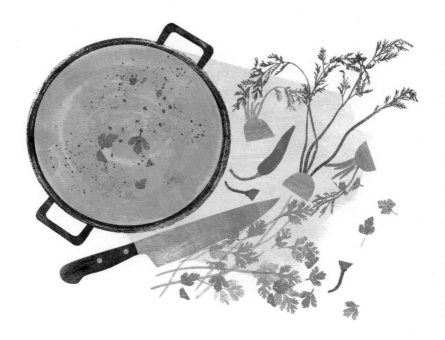

While fruits can be highly nutritious, they can also contain a significant amount of natural sugar, which although naturally occurring, is not helpful for inflammatory conditions when consumed in excess. It may, therefore, be best to stick to a maximum of two to three portions a day, and to avoid those highest in sugar, such as bananas, grapes and especially dried fruit. The best fruits to include are usually dark-coloured berries, which are high in antioxidants and low in sugar.

Omega 3

This type of fatty acid – especially EPA (eicosapentaenoic acid) found in oily fish – is especially important, as it can be converted into substances in the body that help to control inflammation. To get more omega 3, eat oily fish two or three times a week.

Add spice

Spices such as turmeric, ginger and cayenne can be excellent additions to foods because they can have gentle anti-inflammatory properties. Studies have shown that the anti-inflammatory benefits of regular turmeric consumption in food are comparable to over-the-counter non-steroidal anti-inflammatories.

Keep hydrated

Drinking enough water is vital for joint health, as it is for all areas of health. Water helps to remove toxic metabolic waste and dead cells that are produced in higher quantities when there is inflammation, as well as delivering nutrients to the tissues. Try herbal teas, too, such as:

* Nettle tea is high in minerals to support the bones.

* Green tea may be a good source of antioxidants to combat free radicals.

* Rosehip tea has natural anti-inflammatory properties that can be supportive.

* Ginger tea can also be a good option, especially if made using fresh ginger: slice an inch-thick piece and add it to a mug of boiling water – honey and lemon can be added if desired.

Foods to avoid

Sugary foods and refined carbohydrates – Sugar can have a detrimental effect on our health in many ways, including by exacerbating inflammation. Refined carbohydrates – white bread, pastries, pasta, pizza, etc. – break down quickly into sugars when digested, so are just as problematic. Replace these with wholegrain carbohydrates such as brown rice, oats, quinoa and good-quality wholemeal bread. (Some people may do better avoiding wheat altogether and trying rye bread or alternative wheat-free options.) Alcohol is also included in this group. And watch out for added sugar in ultra-processed foods or even foods that are marketed as 'good for you', such as fruity yoghurts and tinned vegetables.

Caffeine – When it comes to tea or coffee, tea is a better option, but stick to one to two cups a day to limit caffeine intake. Try to replace tea and coffee with alternatives such as grain 'coffees' based on barley, rye or chicory, or rooibos tea, which tastes similar to normal tea but is naturally free of caffeine and other stimulating substances.

Red meat and organ meats – These are best limited to one or two servings a week, as they can be acid-forming and high in a pro-inflammatory omega 6 fat called arachidonic acid. They can also be rich in nutrients, however, so for most people they do not need to be excluded entirely.

Fried foods – particularly those fried in vegetable oils. Vegetable oils are high in omega 6 fatty acids, which in high levels can convert to pro-inflammatory substances in the body and also become rancid when heated to high temperatures. Fry or roast food in oil only occasionally. Olive oil is a slightly better alternative to normal vegetable oils, but its fatty acids can still spoil at high temperatures, so avoid heating it to smoking point. Coconut oil is a better alternative because it is mainly composed of saturated fats; it does not spoil at high temperatures, while still providing a healthier alternative to butter and other animal fats. De-odourised coconut oils are available for cooking if you want to avoid the coconut flavour/smell.

Nightshade vegetables – This family of vegetables may cause a problem for those with arthritis, as these foods seem to trigger inflammation in the joints. The nightshade family is tomatoes, white potatoes, aubergine and peppers. (Note: black pepper as a spice is not included in this group and is fine to use.)

🫙 Supplements

Many supplements may be helpful for joint health. As different things may work for different people, it is advisable to choose between one and three of the following types of supplements and try them at the recommended dose for at least three months before judging whether they are going to be helpful or switching to something else.

Multi-nutrient – containing 10mcg of vitamin D, vitamin B12, vitamin C.

Omega 3 – The omega-3 fatty acid EPA (eicosapentaenoic acid) in particular is thought to be the most helpful for reducing inflammation within the joints. Take 1–2g per day.

Glucosamine, MSM and/or chondroitin – These provide the building blocks for cartilage production and repair. 500mg twice a day.

Boswellia – Also known as frankincense, it contains a number of fatty acids and boswellic acid which have anti-inflammatory properties. It has been shown to be especially effective with rheumatoid arthritis. Take 200–400mg 2–3 times daily.

Magnesium oil spray or balm – Magnesium absorbed through the skin may help with pain in the local area.

Turmeric – Research has shown that when turmeric is used in therapeutic doses, it may reduce joint pain and tenderness, cartilage degeneration and joint inflammation. Supplements often focus on just the curcumin content of turmeric, but significant benefits have been found in the turmerosaccharides and turmerone volatile oils within the turmeric root, especially for knee osteoarthritis. Choose a form that provides all of these. Take 1–2g per day. Turmeric and ginger balms have also shown to be effective when applied to the affected area.

 Testing

You may want to consider assessing your vitamin D levels. This can be done through your GP surgery or through a private laboratory.

As a deficiency in omega 3 may also be contributing to your symptoms you can also do a simple pin prick test to check this.

If you are experiencing rheumatoid arthritis, you may want to explore whether a food intolerance or allergy may be contributing to your symptoms. Gluten is a common trigger. However, I suggest that you seek the support of a nutritional therapist or naturopath to make these recommendations and support the results with a plan that is specific to you.

Cholesterol support

An imbalance in cholesterol levels is associated with a number of cardiovascular conditions including atherosclerosis (hardening of the arteries) and therefore a greater risk of heart disease and strokes. Diet and lifestyle plays a significant role in maintaining healthy cholesterol levels.

However, cholesterol, although a significant contributory factor to increased disease risk, is not to be feared. Quite the opposite: cholesterol forms the backbone of many important bodily functions, including protecting cells, transporting hormones and forming the backbone of vitamin D production. The cholesterol that we produce in the body is made by our liver and is fundamental to good health. Some people have a predisposition to produce more of this body-generated cholesterol and therefore will always have a slightly higher cholesterol reading that still may be in the range of 'normal' for them. However, it is when this cholesterol is associated with damaged fats and raised sugar levels from sources in our diet that it becomes an issue.

GETTING TO KNOW CHOLESTEROL

The two main types of cholesterol are high-density cholesterol (HDL), which protects the heart by transporting fats *away* from the arteries, and low-density cholesterol (LDL), which, in higher amounts, has been associated with atherosclerosis. It is the ratio between these two that is important. You will often receive a total cholesterol: HDL score when you are tested. Above 4.5 has been associated with risk of coronary heart disease.

There is another type of fat called triglycerides which, rather than being used to build cells and hormones like cholesterol, is used to store unused calories and provide your body with energy in between meals. High levels of triglycerides may contribute to hardening of the arteries or thickening of the artery walls (arteriosclerosis) – which increases the risk of stroke, heart attack and heart disease. Extremely high triglycerides can also cause acute inflammation of the pancreas (pancreatitis). So understanding your triglyceride levels is equally as important as your cholesterol reading. Some medications can also raise triglycerides:

* Diuretics

* Oestrogen and progesterone medication such as HRT

* Steroids

* Beta blockers

* Some immunosuppressants

PLANT STEROLS

Plant sterols occur naturally in various plant-derived foods, including vegetable oils, such as rapeseed oil and soybean oil, and nuts, grains and seeds. Plant sterols have a very similar structure to cholesterol. This means that when they are eaten, they partially block the uptake of cholesterol from the gastrointestinal tract, thus reducing the cholesterol levels in the bloodstream – particularly the more problematic LDL cholesterol (see box opposite).

There are some commercially available products that have re-synthesised the structure of naturally occurring planet sterols and added these to food, such as spreads. However, getting them from the natural sources, the food of origin, is preferable because it will also contain other cofactors and antioxidants that support a healthy cardiovascular system, as well as needed fibre.

The Mediterranean diet

A Mediterranean-style diet is rich in vegetables, legumes, fruits, wholegrains, nuts, seeds, poultry, fish and olive oil, and it's associated with a lower risk of raised cholesterol, diabetes and heart disease. More recently, researchers have been studying a 'greener' version of the diet, with fewer animal-based and more plant-based proteins (such as nuts and seeds), plus lots of green tea. This shift saw even greater declines in insulin resistance, inflammation markers, cholesterol and blood pressure (Tsaban et al., 2021).

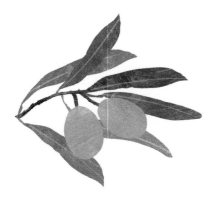

The recommendations in the foundations for a healthy diet in Part One align with many of the principles of the Mediterranean diet. However, here are some areas to pay particular attention to or add.

* **Avoid processed fats and sugars**. Oxidised fats (from diets high in sugar or trans fats, for example) cause damage to healthy cholesterol, make it harder for our body to produce healthy cholesterol and spike triglyceride levels.

* Introduce wholegrains, pulses and vegetables to increase your intake of **natural plant sterols**.

* Eat more red and yellow vegetables and fruit because they are good sources of **vitamin C** and **carotenoids,** which are protective for damaged tissue because of their antioxidant status and also a good source of fibre.

* **High pectin foods** have been shown to be especially effective at removing waste from the gut. Good sources are beetroot, stewed or grated apple or pear and grapefruit. Add them to juices, breakfast and yoghurt or make soups.

* **Vitamin E-rich foods** – Vitamin E protects cholesterol against oxidation and plaque build-up in the arteries. Add at least one portion of avocado, wheatgerm or nuts and nut butters (almond is especially good) to your diet per day. For example, for breakfast or a snack, have nut butter or avocado with lemon juice on toast.

* **Omega 3-rich foods** reduce blood pressure and help to protect healthy cholesterol and arteries. These foods also happen to be good sources of selenium and coenzyme Q10 as well (see page 188). Choose organic where you can.

* 5–10g **soluble fibre** a day decreases total and LDL cholesterol by reducing the absorption into your bloodstream. Good sources include oatmeal, flaxseed, oat bran, barley. Porridge is a great way to eat fibre, as 350g of oats provides 6g of fibre.

* **Turmeric, ginger and garlic** have known effects on supporting the clearance of cholesterol through the liver. Grate ginger into morning breakfast, add garlic to meals (raw is best) or add turmeric root to soups.

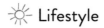 Lifestyle

Look after your beneficial flora
Over 1g of cholesterol is presented to the digestive tract each day.
It is the role of beneficial bacteria to convert at least 200mg of
this into the non-absorbable form of cholesterol. Eating many
of the foods recommended above will support the growth of
beneficial flora. Taking a probiotic supplement or eating small
amounts of fermented foods can also be of significant support.
These include:

* Yoghurt

* Kefir

* Sauerkraut

* Fermented tofu (tempeh)

* Miso

* Fermented apple cider vinegar

Build these into your diet three times per week or as often as you can.
For example, add sauerkraut to cold meats and salad as a pickle, or use
apple cider vinegar in salad dressings or add to hot water and drink.

Exercise regularly
Aim for at least 30 minutes of physical activity on most or all days
of the week. Regular exercise can lower triglycerides and boost
'good' cholesterol. Try to incorporate more physical activity into
your daily tasks – for example, climb the stairs at work or take a
walk during breaks.

STATINS

Statins are prescribed for raised cholesterol levels, but side effects can include muscle pain, nausea and diarrhoea, increased blood sugar levels and therefore a higher risk of type 2 diabetes. They also reduce the body's production of a substance called coenzyme Q10, which our cells use to generate energy and protect themselves from damage. Low levels of coenzyme Q10 have been associated with a greater risk of side effects, specifically muscle pain. Taking additional coenzyme Q10 can reduce some of the side effects, as well as being a natural aid for reducing cholesterol too.

Supplements

Multi-nutrient – containing 10mcg of vitamin D, selenium, vitamin C, vitamin E and the full range of B vitamins.

Omega 3 fatty acids – 1–2g per day.

Broad spectrum probiotic – look for a broad spectrum of strains providing 20–30 billion CFU per dose.

Vitamin B3 – sometimes called niacin or nicotinic acid, can lower your triglycerides and low-density lipoprotein (LDL) cholesterol. Additional supplementation can be useful and doses range from 1,000–2,000mg, starting on a dose of 250mg. However, seek advice specific to you: high doses are not for everyone.

GENERAL HEALTH

When we are generally healthy, it can be so easy to take our bodies for granted. From one season to the next, we forget the inconvenience of suffering minor ailments and can feel surprised and irritated each time cold season rolls around and the whole family is struck down and ill-tempered with each other.

Of course, minor ailments are part of life, but if we follow the principles of wellbeing and ensure we are supporting our bodies with the nutrients they need, then we will know we are doing all we can to ensure they are as short-lived and low impact as possible.

It is always worth remembering that times of stress and insufficient sleep deplete our reserves, and we should therefore take extra care with what nutrients we put into our bodies. If we are going to ask more of ourselves, we need to give ourselves the right level of support and general kindness to make this possible.

Cold and flu

When it comes to seasonal illness, prevention is key. Typically, many of us 'react' to illness – meaning we give our immune system the attention it deserves only when we actually start to feel unwell. This approach isn't the most effective, as building up good levels of nutrients in the body doesn't happen overnight. During or leading up to times of heightened risk of infection, or when our immune system might be particularly susceptible, investing in our immune system's 'armoury' is important.

▽ ☀ Diet and lifestyle

Look after your beneficial flora
Over 70 per cent of the immune system resides in the gut. So eating small amounts of fermented foods and/or taking a probiotic supplement can be of significant support. Probiotic foods should be included in your diet three times per week or as often as you can. They are found naturally in:

* Yoghurt

* Kefir

* Sauerkraut

* Fermented tofu (tempeh)

* Miso

* Fermented apple cider vinegar

Avoid sugar
Sugar is classified as an immuno-suppressant, so if you are keen on sweets, chocolate and cakes, then it's time to consider cutting down so you can allow your immune system to work properly. Remember also that hidden sugars include white bread and pasta and be careful in assuming all 'natural' sugars are fine to consume in higher amounts. For example, dates seem very innocent but are actually very high in fruit sugar. Keep that kind of food as a treat!

Get good sleep
Restorative sleep has a measurable impact on the strength of the immune system. Research has shown that quality sleep is most likely to occur between 10.45pm and 6.45am.

Now scientists understand that getting less sleep leads to an immune system that is under-functioning or even suppressed. Getting enough sleep may enable you to manage inflammatory responses and generally strengthen the immune system. Those finding it hard to fall asleep might consider taking a magnesium supplement before bedtime and drinking valerian tea.

Stress is also unhelpful in connection to the immune system, so look into attempting to cut down or at least manage this long term. Stress may also be better managed with a good night's sleep because we are then able to be more logical and productive during the daytime.

Exercise in the fresh air
Exposure to fresh air has been shown to support the immune system, as has regular exercise. Exercising and walking in the fresh air every day can be beneficial, improving immune defences against bacterial and viral infection. Exercise also reduces stress, which can have a suppressive effect on immune tolerance.

Eat a colourful diet
Getting a wide variety of vitamins, minerals and phytochemicals (natural plant compounds) is essential for good immunity. A recent systematic review found that the immune system is strengthened by good nutrition and should therefore be part of everyday living and any treatment plan to support the immune system for those vulnerable to infections. The colour you see in vegetables and fruit is due to special pigments. These work to support the immune system and provide antioxidant protection when we need it. Think of a rainbow and focus on getting a full spectrum of colour into your daily diet. Fruit and vegetables are also rich in fibre, helping to support gut function, which, again, is pivotal for a healthy immune system.

Eat with the seasons
Nature doesn't make mistakes, and the times of year in which we are more prone to bugs and colds are the winter and autumn

months when we see an abundance of bright berries, such as blackberries, rosehips or elderberries, rich in immune-supporting antioxidants and vitamins C, A and zinc. Eating foods grown in season will help because they are rich in vitamins and minerals that will support your immune system and nourish your body during this time of year.

Have fun
Laughter and community aren't just nice to have – they have been scientifically proven to increase our defences against infection, induce feel-good hormones and reduce stress hormones. So look out for one another and make the most of opportunities to keep the laughter flowing.

Supplements

Natural multi-nutrient – A good-quality multi-nutrient providing vitamin D, zinc, vitamin C, selenium.

Omega 3 oils – providing at least 1,000mg EPA and 750mg DHA. The inflammation moderating effect of omega 3 fatty acids is thought to help prevent colds and flus.

Vitamin D – Epidemiological studies have demonstrated an association between vitamin D deficiency and vulnerability to seasonal influenza. Not everyone will have had a decent amount of summer sun exposure and we can get only around 10 per cent of our required intake from food, so supplementation is recommended. You can take this in addition to your multi-nutrient.

Zinc – Research has shown it can optimise the immune system via its ability to increase white blood cells, which your body needs to fight infection. It also has a crucial role in inhibiting the progression and replication of viruses. It is found in various foods such as seeds and green leafy vegetables, but it is a mineral in which people are commonly low. Your daily multi-nutrient may contain zinc; however, research has shown that up to 30mg of zinc per day at the onset of an upper respiratory tract infection can reduce symptoms and the time of illness significantly.

Vitamin C – supports a healthy immune system and contributes to protecting against infection. Fruit and vegetables are by far the best sources. However, vitamin C must be consistently topped up because it cannot be manufactured by the body when there is need to support healing. Research has shown that food and natural nutrients that use the Food-Grown® philosophy to produce vitamin C (when supplemented) are more effective and better retained by the body for longer, in comparison to synthetic versions (see page 25 for more on Food-Grown® supplements). You may be able to find this within your daily multi-nutrient. If not, take 60mg of natural vitamin C per day. You can increase this amount to 300mg when experiencing the onset of sniffles, to reduce the severity of symptoms.

Medicinal mushrooms – such as maitake and oyster mushrooms are rich in active compounds called polysaccharides, the most well-researched of which are beta glucan 1-3 and beta glucan 1-6. These molecules have been shown to support the immune system's response to viral and bacterial infection.

Elderberry – has the ability to inhibit several strains of the flu virus. It can reduce the duration of flu symptoms by increasing the antibody level to combat flu and help fight off the illness. This wonderful botanical also seems to reduce inflammation, which could explain why it has a pronounced effect on reducing aches, pain and fever. You can buy it in a syrup or make your own.

NAC – the antioxidant N-acetyl-L-cysteine (NAC) has been shown to inhibit the replication of seasonal human influenza A viruses.

Turmeric – 'spice of life' turmeric/curcumin has been used for thousands of years in traditional medicine. The diverse range of health benefits of turmeric are linked to its multi-target activity in the body, and include immune modulation, antiviral, anti-inflammatory, antioxidant and anti-microbial properties. Curcumin, the naturally occurring compound within the turmeric root, has been much studied, but using the whole root or supplements containing the full spectrum of curcuminoids allows for better synergy and a wider array of benefits. Full spectrum turmeric products and the fresh root also contain small amounts of volatile turmeric essential oil that enhance bioavailability and absorption.

Hay fever

Hay fever, or seasonal allergies, range from being a slight nuisance to a real disruption to daily life. This is a guide to surviving the hay fever season, but it is worth applying this information throughout the year. Supporting the immune system over the long term may help reduce sensitivity in following years.

Those who experience seasonal allergies are classified under the broad medical category of being 'atopic'. This means they have a predisposition towards developing certain allergic hypersensitivity reactions. Simple dietary and lifestyle changes may support sufferers' sensitivity and you can apply the advice here to other atopic conditions such as eczema or asthma.

Histamine is a substance released by the immune system in response to stimuli or substances that the body is allergic or intolerant to, and this is why we experience unpleasant symptoms such as:

* Itchy eyes

* Runny nose

* Itchy skin

* Headache or brain fog

Histamine travels through our bloodstream; therefore, it has contact with all our organs and systems.

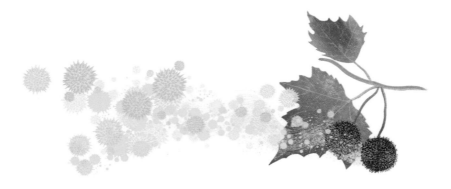

HAY FEVER ALLERGENS

Hay fever symptoms vary from month to month and can last from February to October. Here are the common allergens, and when you're likely to be most affected by them:

February–May	Hazel, elder, birch pollen
April, May	Plane tree pollen
June–August	Grass pollen
August–October	Mould and fungal spores in damp weather

 Diet and lifestyle

Alcohol
Those with atopic type conditions like seasonal allergies may wish to trial cutting down on alcohol to see if symptoms lessen. Grapes grown for wine can often contain lots of pesticides and during the wine production process sulphates are added, to which some people are intolerant. Generally speaking, attempt to cut down on alcohol and if you do want to have a drink, look for an organic wine that is sulphate free, or swap wine for a moderate amount of vodka or gin and tonic instead.

It may be beneficial to consider a gentle cleansing programme where all alcohol is avoided, but do follow a healthy eating plan before and during taking this step so that your liver has the right nutrients in order to detoxify safely and effectively. I recommend seeking the advice of a nutritional therapist or naturopath to support you with this.

Bring in the rainbow
Vegetables and fruits are high in vitamin C, which is essential for immune function and as a natural antihistamine. Each 'colour' within a vegetable or fruit provides a different array of natural anti-inflammatory chemicals called phytochemicals, such as flavonoids. Other plant antioxidants such as carotenoids, polyphenols and bioflavonoids have been found to offer immune-supporting benefits and specific research has gone into a plant compound called anthocyanins. These are more commonly found in red-purple fruit and vegetables such as:

* Blueberries
* Elderberry
* Red cabbage
* Beetroot

I recommend aiming for five to seven servings (a dessertspoon size) of mixed coloured vegetables per day. Remember – as many different colours as possible!

Cook with spices
Spices such as turmeric, ginger and cayenne can be excellent additions to foods, as they can have gentle anti-inflammatory properties. Red onions and garlic are also effective against excess histamine.

Feed your gut

As we know, a large proportion of the immune system is present in our gut. It is important, therefore, to help beneficial bacteria flourish by ingesting probiotic foods or supplements that contain so-called 'good' bacteria, such as bifidobacteria and lactobacillus species, and by consuming foods high in soluble fibre that good bugs like to eat, called prebiotics.

Probiotics are beneficial microorganisms found in the gut which are also called friendly bacteria and can be helpful in re-inoculating the gut. Note that taking antibiotics kills both good and bad bacteria. Probiotic powders are versatile and argued by some experts to be more effectively utilised by the body in a free powder or liquid form.

As more is understood about the complexity of the human microbiome, we are also recognising that strains of beneficial flora work best in synergy. Look for complexes with multiple strains, such as those containing lactobacillus, bifidobacterium and streptococcus strains, which have been shown to be beneficial for hay fever and seasonal allergies specifically.

Prebiotics are non-digestible food ingredients that selectively stimulate the growth of beneficial microorganisms already in the colon. In other words, prebiotics feed probiotics. Prebiotics are available in many foods that contain a fibre called inulin, including:

* Artichokes

* Garlic

* Shiitake mushrooms

* Leeks

* Onion

* Rocket

* Chicory

* Edamame beans
* Grains such as barley, flax, oats and sourdough bread

Prioritise certain nutrients:

Zinc – Many people commonly have insufficient blood levels of zinc (although it's not routinely tested by GPs), which may be unhelpful long term if that person is also prone to seasonal allergies. Zinc may inhibit the production of histamine and while nuts, seeds and vegetables are good sources, don't forget that seafood and meat are also excellent too.

Omega-3 fatty acids – EPA (eicosapentaenoic acid) found in oily fish in particular can be converted into substances in the body which help to control inflammation. To get more omega 3, eat oily fish such as sardines, mackerel, trout and salmon two or three times a week. Include omega-3-rich seeds – flaxseeds and chia seeds – and cold-pressed oils of these seeds in your diet. Other seeds and raw nuts are rich in omega 6 essential fatty acids and also contain some omega 3.

Bee products – consuming bee pollen has traditionally been used for seasonal allergies, but research is now showing the benefits too. Thousands of people swear that a spoonful of local honey daily, preferably starting well before the pollen season, has transformed their lives as far as hay fever is concerned. There's no real evidence either way, but for some people it really does seem to work. The principle behind it is desensitisation – the pollen that bees collect is the heavy-grained variety that doesn't cause problems and appears to work well as an effective anti-allergen.

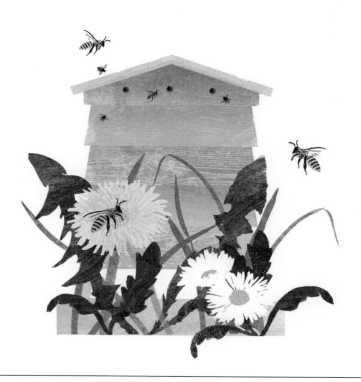

🫙 Supplements

B vitamins such as B6 – These are helpful for managing histamine production – as is increasing your intake of vegetables and meat to access a good source of B vitamins (although look for free range and ideally organic meat).

Vitamin C and bioflavonoids (especially quercetin) – These are natural antihistamines, so it can be beneficial to build foods rich in these, such as citrus fruits, onions, garlic and parsley, into your diet at least six weeks before the onset of your usual annual symptoms.

Remember that humans cannot manufacture vitamin C and anyone who is experiencing immune sensitivity issues should make sure they keep their levels topped up. Much research has shown that select flavonoids possess anti-allergic, anti-inflammatory, antiviral and antioxidant activities. Both vitamin C and bioflavonoids are key nutrients to consider for hay fever support because they have been shown to inhibit histamine release. You may need to take up to 3g daily for beneficial effects. Combine with quercetin to balance histamine levels and enhance the actions of vitamin C. Bromelain is an enzyme found in fruits such as pineapple and although it has less robust research than vitamin C or quercetin, it has been shown to support healthy nasal and respiratory airways and may help to increase absorption of quercetin.

 Testing

You may want to explore whether a food intolerance or allergy may be contributing to your symptoms. Gluten is a common trigger. However, I suggest that you seek the support of a nutritional therapist or naturopath to make these recommendations and support the results with a plan that is specific to you.

As a deficiency in omega 3 may also be contributing to your symptoms, you can also do a simple pin prick test to check this too.

WOMEN'S HEALTH

When we talk about women's health, what we are actually talking about is hormonal health in women, and there is no greater illustration of the interconnection and sophisticated nature of our health than this.

The hormones that support female reproductive and menstrual health are part of the endocrine system, and it is like a large orchestra. There are many different hormones, or instruments, that need to play in balance to create harmony. When one is out of tune, it affects the whole performance. Having the right instruments, playing at the right time, is conducted by your brain. Feeding your body the right tools – not only to create these instruments but to play them at the right time and in the right amounts – is a fundamental part of hormonal balance. But as you will see, what is important is not only what you are (or are not) putting into your body, but also how well you are sleeping and moving, and your stress and mood. You will also discover that what you put on your body matters too, with certain environmental toxins influencing your hormonal harmony.

Hormonal conditions are complex, but you will notice that many of the recommendations to support them are the same; this is because many of the underlying influences are shared. You will find that those experiencing PMS, polycystic ovary syndrome (PCOS) and fibroids all benefit from additional omega 3 and building in colour into their food choices; perimenopause, menopause, endometriosis and adenomyosis all benefit from adding in more pulses and phytoestrogen rich foods; and all of them benefit from supporting our experience of stress, sleep and the way we move.

At the heart of many of the topics in this section is oestrogen: a key instrument within our hormonal orchestra. Oestrogen plays an important role in the normal sexual and reproductive development of women from the early to middle years of our lives, but it also has other important functions in the body. It supports brain function by protecting nerve endings and the areas in the brain responsible for cognition and memory; promotes bone formation by supporting the activity of cells known as osteoblasts to make new bone; and protects the muscles of the heart and blood vessels, as well as controlling cholesterol levels and the build-up of fat in the arteries.

It is also worth being mindful of environmental oestrogens that may act as harmful hormone disruptors. For women with endometriosis, xenoestrogens can pose a threat to hormonal stability. Xenoestrogens are industrial compounds found in the man-made environment, such as in the chemicals used to make plastic or bleaching agents, which structurally mimic oestrogen and elicit an 'oestrogenic' affect in the body. To minimise these, don't cook or heat foods in plastic – use glass or crockery instead. Use pots or frying pans made of steel or non-toxic cookware. Minimise use of chemical-based cosmetics and household cleaning products. Smoking can lead to the earlier onset of the menopause, so if you are a smoker, consider giving up. A supported nutritional programme to support your body in metabolising a build-up of toxic material can be helpful, including that generated by high stress or a compromised diet over the years. Seek the support of a nutritional therapist or naturopath to do this.

Endometriosis and adenomyosis

Endometriosis is a complex disorder of the female reproductive tract, whereby cells similar to those found in the lining of the womb are found elsewhere in the body. During the female monthly cycle, the fluctuation in hormones stimulates these cells to grow, then break down and bleed, as they would in the lining of the womb, leading to inflammation, pain and the formation of scar tissue. Endometriosis is one of the most common gynaecological conditions and it is estimated that approximately 10–15 per cent of all premenopausal women have endometriosis, but despite its prevalence, it is still underdiagnosed, taking approximately 7½ years for some women to get a diagnosis.

Adenomyosis is similar to endometriosis but endometrial deposits are found nestled within the muscle fibres of the wall of the womb itself. These form diffuse patches or lumps similar to fibroids.

How endometriosis and adenomyosis occur remains controversial. One of the most supported theories is that endometriosis is fuelled by a relative dominance of the hormone oestrogen, but growing research suggests that there is an autoimmune aspect to the condition.

Studies have demonstrated that nutritional therapy (diet and supplements) is a more effective approach in terms of pain relief and improving quality of life post-surgery than medical hormonal treatment. Women with endometriosis statistically have low levels of vitamin D, zinc, omega 3 and vitamin A. Nutrient deficiencies come about as a result of not enough food or too much of the wrong food. Sometimes it can be that we are eating well but not well enough to provide the specific nutrients we need to heal from a specific condition.

Endometriosis and adenomyosis are complex conditions and although the recommendations below are an excellent starting point, I highly recommend further reading on nutrition and endometriosis or seeking a nutritional therapist or naturopath.

▽ ☼ Diet and lifestyle

Some gentle changes really can help you make strides in your experience of endometriosis.

Eat colour
Research shows that women who eat green vegetables 13 times or more per week (roughly twice a day) are 70 per cent less likely to

develop endometriosis. One study concluded that carotenoid-rich foods (especially citrus fruit) also positively affected symptoms of endometriosis (Harris et al., 2018). Use smoothies, juicing or soups to deeply nourish.

Befriend your gut
Beneficial gut bacteria can reduce the production of beta-glucuronidase, an enzyme that can prevent oestrogen from being removed from the gut and instead recirculates it in the bloodstream. Incorporate natural, organic yoghurt into your daily diet, either on its own or in dressings and sauces. Fermented foods such as sauerkraut or kefir are excellent sources of beneficial bacteria too or take a probiotic supplement (minimum 10 billion CFU).

Keep up your minerals
Abundant amounts of zinc and magnesium are used up during states of physical imbalance. During menstruation, women can lose up to half their magnesium supply. Women with endometriosis and adenomyosis often suffer from heavy bleeding during a period and this significantly reduces their stores of the mineral iron.

Be conscious of what you put in and on your body
Non-organic tampons use bleached paper products that contain dioxins, proven to have an adverse effect on the hormonal system. You can find more information from the Women's Environmental Network (www.wen.org.uk).

Consider your gluten intake
More recently, research that has categorised endometriosis as an autoimmune condition has documented an improved response in those following a gluten-free diet: 75 per cent of participants found a significant decrease in symptoms when they cut out gluten over 12 months (Marziali et al., 2012).

Eat phytoestrogen-rich foods

Phytoestrogens are plant hormones with a similar structure to human oestrogens; they have the ability to lower oestrogen levels when they are too high and increase them if they are too low. They are found in flax, wholegrains and fermented soya such as fermented tofu and tempeh. They have been shown to have the added benefit of being protective for heart health too.

Build in cruciferous vegetables

Cauliflower, cabbage, kale, pak choi, broccoli, Brussels sprouts, mustard plant and rocket all contain naturally occurring plant compounds called indoles, which support oestrogen processing.

Essential fats

Oily fish (omega 3) helps to increase beneficial oestrogens and remove the more rogue breakdown products when oestrogen is metabolised, as well as moderate levels of inflammation. More recent research is discovering a link between levels of inflammation in the body and hormone imbalance.

Stress management

Glands and organs required to stabilise stress are also key manufacturing sites for hormones, including oestrogen, progesterone and testosterone. This means that there is less available to produce these hormones. Stress hormones also affect the efficiency with which we process and remove hormones through the liver and gut once we've used them. This can lead to higher amounts of rogue forms of oestrogen, tipping the balance further. Additionally, stress increases nutrient demands in the body and can change our behaviour around food – for example, making us more reliant on quick fixes. But sugar, caffeine and alcohol destabilise blood sugar balance, initiating a stress response, as well as blocking enzymes that help the body to clear used oestrogen. Zinc and magnesium are used up quickly in periods of physical and mental stress – as endometriosis is a state of physical stress, the demand for these nutrients is even greater than normal. During particularly stressful times and during menstruation, women can lose up to half their magnesium supply.

Supplements

Multi-nutrient for your life stage – Look for one that contains 5–10mg zinc for testosterone, 10mg B6 for energy and hormone regulation, and 5–10mcg vitamin D, as this can help regulate sex hormones.

Magnesium – 84 per cent of patients with dysmenorrhoea (painful periods) reported a decline in symptoms after supplementing with magnesium. Take 80mg of Food-Grown® magnesium or 400mg of synthetic alternative. Magnesium balms and oils can be supportive too, as can magnesium bath salts. Take at night.

Vitamin B6 – is required for the healthy clearance and production of oestrogen and has been shown to be beneficial in endometriosis. Look to have this included in your multi-nutrient, but you also may benefit from additional vitamin B6.

Omega 3 – A study of teens with endometriosis reported a 50 per cent decrease in pain scores when supplementing with omega 3. Take 1,000mg per day.

Iron – if you are experiencing heavy blood loss and clotting, take 10–14mg of natural Food-Grown® iron to reduce nausea and digestive side effects.

Turmeric – research shows turmeric works as an anti-inflammatory, reducing the severity and progression of endometriosis lesions. It has also been shown to be a potent antispasmodic when taken two weeks before menstruation. Supplements often focus on the curcumin content of turmeric, but significant benefits have been found in the turmerosaccharides and turmerone volatile oils within the turmeric root. Choose a form that provides all of these. Take 1–2g per day. Turmeric balms have also shown to be effective to rub on areas of cramping.

The amino acid methionine and the herbs dong quai, agnus castus, milk thistle and dandelion have also been shown to be especially beneficial. Look for a supplement designed to specifically support endometriosis which includes these. I also recommend consulting a herbal practitioner for advice on herbs that might be suitable specific to you.

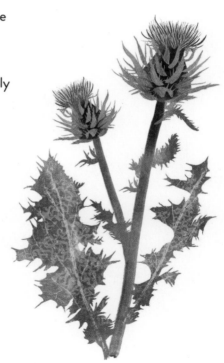

Menstrual imbalances

Premenstrual syndrome (PMS) or premenstrual tension (PMT), is a recurrent condition characterised by troublesome symptoms usually 7–14 days prior to menstruating. Typical symptoms are decreased energy, tension, irritability, depression, headache, change to libido, breast pain, back pain, bloating and/or water retention. Although the range of symptoms is wide, the underlying hormonal patterns in PMS are common – often an imbalance of the ratio of oestrogen and progesterone.

Other menstrual disorders that are caused or impacted by hormone imbalances include:

* **Dysmenorrhea** – painful cramping during menstruations, sometimes including blood clots.

* **Menorrhagia** – heavy or prolonged menstrual bleeding, commonly including heavy blood clots.

* **Amenorrhea** – the absence of menstruation, often defined as missing one or more menstrual periods. If menstruation has not started before the age of 15 this is known as primary amenorrhea.

Dysmenorrhea and menorrhagia are associated with conditions including endometriosis and polycystic ovary syndrome (PCOS – see pages 170–75). Amenorrhea can be associated with disordered eating patterns and PCOS. If you are missing periods or suffering heavy periods, seek support to investigate if there are any underlying condition such as PCOS, endometriosis or fibroids.

Bear in mind that changes to diet or supplementation are generally thought to take up to three months or three cycles to properly take effect.

▽ ☀ Diet and lifestyle

Studies have shown that women who consume more dairy products and refined carbohydrates – which are lower in nutrients and higher in fast-releasing sugars – experienced greater symptoms of PMS. These women were also shown to be lower in key minerals, including iron, zinc and manganese. There is no doubt that diet plays a part in PMS, so it is worth considering this carefully.

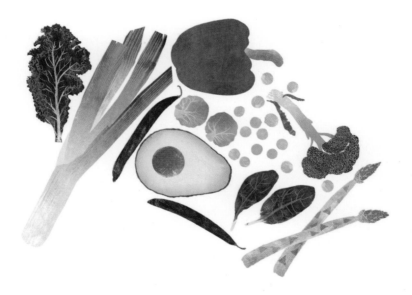

Eat plenty of fruit and veg
Research has shown that women who eat green vegetables 13 times or more per week (roughly twice a day) benefit from greater hormonal balance and the reduction of symptoms associated with menstrual imbalance. Carotenoid-rich foods, especially citrus fruits, were found to have similar benefits.

Look after your beneficial gut bacteria
The 'good' gut bacteria can reduce the production of beta-glucuronidase, an enzyme that remakes oestrogen in the gut and can contribute to its dominance. Incorporate natural, organic yoghurt into your daily diet for a food source of good bacteria, either on its own or in dressings and sauces. Fermented foods such as sauerkraut or kefir are excellent sources of beneficial bacteria too, or take a probiotic supplement (minimum 10 billion CFU).

Reduce your caffeine intake
Studies have shown an incremental increase in the symptoms of PMS related to increased caffeine consumption. Not only does it affect blood sugar levels but it also has a diuretic effect, which can increase the elimination of minerals such as zinc and iron.

Phytoestrogen-rich foods
Phytoestrogens are plant hormones with a similar structure to human oestrogens but they have the ability to lower oestrogen levels when they are too high and increase them if they are too low. Try flax, wholegrains and fermented soya such as fermented tofu and tempeh. They have been shown to have the added benefit of being protective for heart health too.

Essential fats
Oily fish (omega 3) helps to increase beneficial oestrogens, decrease harmful oestrogen metabolites and moderate inflammation. More recent research is discovering a link between levels of inflammation in the body and hormone imbalance to provide essential fats to reduce inflammation.

Stress management
The glands and organs required to stabilise stress are also key manufacturing sites for hormones, including oestrogen, progesterone and testosterone. This means that when you are

stressed their capacity to produce these hormones is reduced, which can exacerbate the erratic nature of them further. Stress hormones also affect the efficiency with which we process and remove hormones through the liver and gut once we've used them. This can lead to higher amounts of rogue forms of oestrogen, tipping the balance further. Additionally, stress increases nutrient demands in the body and can change our behaviour around food – for example, making us more reliant on quick fixes. But sugar, caffeine and alcohol destabilise blood sugar balance, initiating a stress response, as well as blocking enzymes that help the body to clear used oestrogen.

Supplements

Multi-nutrient for your life stage – Look for 5–10mg zinc for testosterone regulation, 10mg B6 for energy and hormone regulation, plus 5–10mcg vitamin D to regulate sex hormones.

Evening primrose oil or starflower oil – both contain gamma linoleic acid or GLA, which has been shown to be effective in reducing breast pain and tenderness associated with PMS. Take 240mg of GLA per day.

Magnesium – 84 per cent of patients with dysmenorrhoea (painful periods) reported a decline in symptoms after taking magnesium. Take 80mg of Food-Grown® magnesium or 400mg of synthetic alternative. Magnesium balms and oils can be supportive too as can magnesium bath salts. Take at night.

Vitamin B6 – is required for the healthy clearance and production of oestrogen. Look to have this included in your multi-nutrient, but you also may benefit from additional vitamin B6.

Omega 3 – Take 1,000mg of omega 3 a day. Studies have shown a significant decrease in pain and cramping (dysmenorrhea) when supplementing with omega 3.

The amino acid methionine, the herbs dong quai, St John's wort, agnus castus or chaste berry, milk thistle and dandelion have also been shown to be especially beneficial to those suffering menstrual disorders. Look for a supplement designed to support PMS specifically which includes these. I also recommend consulting a herbal practitioner for advice on herbs that might be suitable specific to you.

PCOS

Polycystic ovary syndrome develops for many different reasons, some of which are not yet fully understood, though it is thought it affects between 5 and 10 per cent of women. What is known is that women with PCOS produce higher levels of a group of hormones called androgens, the primary of which is testosterone. It is thought that this excess is produced by both the adrenal glands and the ovaries and is both affected by and causes imbalances in insulin, a pivotal hormone for blood sugar management. It is also thought that PCOS is genetic and women with a family history of diabetes may have a higher risk of developing the condition.

These imbalances in both androgens and insulin can result in symptoms including an irregular menstrual cycle, acne, body hair, weight management issues, mood changes and reduced ovulation or anovulation (when periods stop). Some women experience a number or a few of these symptoms and are diagnosed with PCOS. However, some women do not experience any of the symptoms but still present with polycystic ovaries and in these cases would be diagnosed as having polycystic ovaries (small fluid-filled sacs on the ovaries).

PCOS is a complex condition involving multiple systems in the body and therefore requires holistic support, with diet and exercise playing a crucial role in any treatment plan. A supportive diet for someone with PCOS is one low in grains, high glycaemic foods, refined sugar and trans fats, and rich in fibre from a variety of vegetables and pulses, as well as nourishing fats from seeds, nuts, olive oil and avocados. Good blood sugar management is particularly vital and there is now a robust body of evidence which suggests that reducing your intake of sugars and grains can improve management of PCOS. Trying to limit your exposure to synthetic compounds that interact with hormone receptors, whether environmental, dietary or from toiletries, can also be helpful.

There is evidence to suggest that the health of the digestive system, detoxification efficiency and sub- or hyper-functioning of the thyroid can also influence the development and progression of PCOS. Our exposure to and management of stress can also be greatly influential, and finding the right support to help you find more balance and time to pause in your daily life is crucial, whether that is through gentle massage, reading, music or spending time in nature as often as you can. Regularly exercising in nature in a way that suits you and your lifestyle improves your body's production of sex hormone-binding globulin (SHBG), which helps to regulate oestrogen and testosterone, as well as supporting mood, stress and balancing weight.

Deficiencies in certain nutrients such as B vitamins (inositol especially – see the nutrition section over the page), chromium and vitamin D have also been shown to influence PCOS, and supplementing can be supportive.

Maintaining a healthy weight is especially important. Adipose tissue that develops as fat produces a drip feed of hormones that can further disrupt the hormonal imbalance at the centre of PCOS. Being overweight can also further disrupt the body's sensitivity to insulin, thereby increasing the risk of developing type 2 diabetes. Some studies have shown that women with PCOS can benefit from following an intermittent fasting regime to support glucose regulation and weight management.

▽ ☀ Diet and lifestyle

Diet has been shown to help restore a hormonal imbalance that may be contributing to the development or growth of fibroids, as well as supporting nutrient deficiencies that can occur because of heavy blood loss or clotting. PCOS is a condition involving low-level chronic inflammation and therefore following a diet with the following will support this too.

Vitamin D-rich foods
Vitamin D may help reduce your risk of developing fibroids by up to 32 per cent. Include eggs, liver and oily fish – such as salmon, sardines, herring and mackerel – into your weekly diet. Exercise regularly outside to expose yourself to sunlight.

Essential fats
Essential fats found in nuts, seeds, avocado, fish, flax oil and olive oil can be especially supportive in moderating hormone imbalances and supporting skin health and blood sugar regulation. Oily fish (omega 3) helps to increase beneficial oestrogens, decrease harmful oestrogen metabolites and moderate inflammation.

Feed your gut
Foods which feed beneficial gut bacteria are known as prebiotics and good sources of these are fermented foods such as sauerkraut or kimchi, as well as chicory, artichokes, garlic oats, leeks, apples and pears. They help the body to process oestrogen correctly.

Phytoestrogen-rich foods
Phytoestrogens are plant hormones with a similar structure to human oestrogens but have the ability to lower oestrogen levels when they are too high and increase them if they are too low. Try flax, wholegrains and fermented soya such as fermented tofu. They have been shown to have the added benefit of being protective for heart health too.

Fibre-rich foods
Build foods high in fibre into your diet, such as green vegetables, pumpkin, sunflower and sesame seeds and wholegrains. These provide B vitamins such as vitamin B6 and magnesium as hormone building blocks.

Stress management
Glands and organs required to stabilise stress are also key manufacturing sites for hormones including oestrogen, progesterone and testosterone. This means that their capacity to produce these hormones is reduced, which can exacerbate the erratic nature of them further. Stress hormones also affect the efficiency with which we process and remove hormones through the liver and gut once we've used them. This can lead to higher amounts of rogue forms of oestrogen, tipping the balance further. Additionally stress increases nutrient demands in the body and can change our behaviour around food – making us more reliant on quick fixes.

Reduce sugar, caffeine and alcohol intake
Sugar, caffeine and alcohol all make blood sugar balance irregular
and initiate a stress response, as well as block enzymes that help
the body to clear oestrogen. Zinc and magnesium are used up in
abundant amounts during states of physical and mental stress.

Build in protein
Protein is also a source of alpha-lipoic acid and coenzyme Q10, plus
magnesium and B vitamins needed for energy production. As well as
magnesium, B vitamins are essential for blood sugar regulation and
normal hormone function.

Good sources of protein include foods such as:

* Meat

* Fish

* Nuts

* Seeds

* Beans / lentils

* Eggs

🫙 Supplements

Multi-nutrient for your life stage – This should include 5–10mg
zinc to help regulate testosterone, 10mg vitamin B6 for energy
and hormone regulation, chromium for blood sugar regulation, and
5–10mcg vitamin D to help regulate sex hormones.

Vitamin D – Have your vitamin D levels measured and if found to be low top up your multi-nutrient with 10mcg of vitamin D. Reassess after three months.

B vitamin complex – B vitamins are recommended for women with PCOS to regulate hormone balance, especially B6, folate and B12. If you are taking metformin to treat type 2 diabetes, then it is especially important to take B12.

Inositol – This is a member of the B vitamin family and is found in beans, nuts, meat and most grains and has been shown to improve insulin resistance and aid weight management. It is sometimes combined with alpha lipoic acid or coenzyme Q10 to improve this action further, although inositol in isolation is very effective. Take 1–2g per day.

Perimenopause and menopause

Menopause is a natural, transitionary stage, moving a woman away from the child-bearing years into a stage that, according to Ayurvedic and traditional Chinese medicine, is characterised by 'soul development'. A Native American saying tells us: 'At her first period a girl meets her wisdom. Through her menstruating years she practices her wisdom, and at menopause she becomes her wisdom.'

Perimenopause is defined as the time leading up to the menopause and can begin up to ten years before menopause occurs. It is when oestrogen, progesterone and testosterone levels rise and fall erratically, as the ovaries prepare to stop releasing eggs entirely, slowing down the reproductive system until one reaches the menopause. Just like puberty, it marks a significant hormonal transition for the body. Strictly speaking, full menopause is only one day – it is the day after the absence of a menstrual period for more than one year. This usually occurs between the ages 45 and 55, with the average age being 51 years in the UK. The time after this period is known as post-menopause.

Until recently, perimenopause was mistakenly lumped in with menopause, rather than understood as its own life stage. Menopause was often thought of as hot flushes and night sweats only, which left women unaware of the more than 48 symptoms associated with perimenopause. This may be why, although half the population will experience it, two out of three women find themselves blindsided by it. It is not uncommon for women to be wrongly diagnosed with depression, burnout or anxiety in the lead-up to menopause, as many of the symptoms overlap. In fact, statistics have shown that 90 per cent of women don't recognise the immediate link to their fluctuating and declining hormones, instead attributing symptoms to ageing, stress, anxiety or depression (Wild Nutrition, 2022). This may be starting to change as awareness increases, but studies have shown that in the UK, women need to visit their GP six times on average before their symptoms are correctly attributed to the perimenopause.

Symptoms can be physical, mental and social – from erratic periods, sleep issues and headaches to mood swings, drops in libido, memory lapses and anxiety, as well as dryness of the skin, vagina and/or hair. Women moving into perimenopause may experience almost PMS-type symptoms rather than classic menopause symptoms – which are often confused. Vasomotor symptoms are more commonly referred to as 'hot flushes' or 'night sweats'. Women may experience often rapid changes in body temperature, palpitations and a shift between experiencing heat and chills. It is thought that the hypothalamus (which controls body temperature) is affected by changes in the levels of oestradiol (the most potent form of oestrogen) and the hormone LH.

Women should seek advice as soon as they begin to see changes in their cycle. Perimenopause can go on for some time, but only a professional will be able to support deciphering the difference between perimenopause and other conditions like PMS or mild depression. A nutritional therapist may also recommend some hormone testing, either through a GP or privately. Some changes in cycle and symptoms may be better managed naturally if dealt with earlier on. Very often, women who are very tired, stressed and overworked will find perimenopause a challenge. Supporting the adrenal glands and energy systems should begin early.

Whatever a woman's experience, it is vitally important to remember that this is not a disease, it is a natural progression to a different stage of a woman's life cycle and that it is a mind, body and spirit experience. I sometimes explain perimenopause as being a plane that is coming into land, with menopause being the airport. How bumpy this journey is will be strongly impacted by your nutritional and emotional wellbeing during this time. Proactively caring for yourself and the body systems that are being affected by changes in hormone levels is the best strategy if this ebb and flow is to be experienced as a positive transition.

▽ ☼ Diet and lifestyle

As the impact and severity of symptoms will be determined or at least influenced by your diet and lifestyle, there is much you can do to support your body before, during and after this time to make your experience more manageable – just like preparing for a marathon. Investing in self-care through a wholesome diet, stress management and exercise is important. Just like any other important life transition, such as pregnancy or puberty, you may need to change things to support yourself while you are going through this stage.

Try phytoestrogen-rich foods
Phytoestrogens are plant hormones with a similar structure to human oestrogens but have the ability to lower oestrogen levels when they are too high and increase them if they are too low. Try flax, wholegrains, fermented soya such as fermented tofu. They have been shown to have the added benefit of being protective for heart health too.

Eat enough protein
It is important to eat enough protein during this life stage; we need bones and muscle mass to support the structure around our joints, but also to fortify our skin, promote healthy detoxification and balance our mood, hormones and blood sugar levels.

Enjoy fibre-rich foods
Make sure that you have enough fibre-rich foods, such as green vegetables, pumpkin, sunflower and sesame seeds and wholegrains. These provide B vitamins such as vitamin B6 and magnesium, which are hormone building blocks that also support gut health.

Build in cruciferous vegetables
Cauliflower, cabbage, kale, pak choi, broccoli, Brussels sprouts, mustard plant and rocket all contain indoles which support oestrogen processing.

Feed your gut
Build in foods that promote the growth of helpful bacteria in the gut. These foods are known as prebiotics and good sources are fermented foods such as sauerkraut or kimchi, as well as chicory, artichokes, garlic, oats, leeks, apples and pears. They help the body to process oestrogen correctly. Poor balance of bacteria in the gut also leads to bloating and distension, common symptoms of menopause, so prebiotics will help address this too.

Embrace essential fats

Essential fats found in nuts, seeds, avocado, fish, flax oil and olive oil can be especially supportive in moderating hormone imbalances, promoting skin health and alleviating symptoms associated with menopause, such as joint pain and vaginal dryness. Oily fish (omega 3) helps to increase beneficial oestrogens, decrease harmful oestrogen metabolites and moderate inflammation. More recently, research has been looking at the role that inflammation could play in exacerbating the symptoms associated with perimenopause and menopause, and whether essential fatty acids including DHA and EPA may help to reduce them.

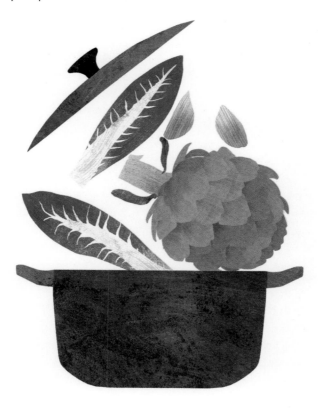

Prioritise stress management

Perimenopause tends to hit at a time when demands on women are often high: career, looking after children and sometimes increasing responsibility for ageing parents. The glands and organs required to stabilise stress are also key manufacturing sites for hormones including oestrogen, progesterone and testosterone. This means that there are less resources available within the body to produce these hormones, which can exacerbate the increasingly erratic nature of them further. Stress hormones also affect the efficiency with which we process and remove hormones through the liver and gut once we've used them. This can lead to higher amounts of oestrogen, tipping the balance further. Additionally, stress increases nutrient demands in the body and can change our behaviour around food – for example, making us more reliant on quick fixes like sugar and caffeine, which we may use as a pick-me-up. Reducing sugar, caffeine and alcohol, which make blood sugar balance irregular and initiate a stress response, as well as blocking enzymes that help the body to clear oestrogen, often provides beneficial results in the longer term. Prioritising whatever stress-reducing techniques work for you is very important at this time.

Practise daily stillness

This stage in life can be the opportunity to take an audit of our life – physically, mentally, emotionally, spiritually – and some women find that in this time, they have a greater sense of self-awareness and a desire to make some changes or do things differently. Adopting a few moments of stillness or quiet on a daily basis can help us to reflect on where we are in our life.

Get good sleep

There is a direct link between the quality of our sleep and hormone regulation. Sleep can also be affected by the change in hormones (progesterone primarily) and adopting some of the recommendations in the section on sleep (see pages 109–11) may well be highly beneficial.

Look at your environment
Be mindful of environmental oestrogens that may act as harmful hormone disruptors. To minimise these, don't cook or heat foods in plastic – use glass or crockery instead. Use pots or frying pans made of steel or non-toxic cookware. Minimise use of chemical-based cosmetics and household cleaning products. Smoking can lead to earlier onset of the menopause, so if you are a smoker, consider giving up. A nutritional programme targeted to support your body in metabolising a build-up of toxic material can be helpful, including that generated by high stress or a compromised diet over the years. Seek the support of a nutritional therapist or naturopath to do this, who will be able to tailor it to meet your requirements and circumstances.

Establish a healthy weight
If you struggle in this area, it's worth knowing that hypo- and hyperthyroidism can affect menopause and perimenopause symptoms, so you may also want to check this with your GP. If you haven't always had the easiest relationship with food, then addressing your diet with a view to losing weight can feel difficult or intimidating. You can get support to do this and should never feel ashamed to ask. For all of us, reviewing our eating habits and focusing on good ways to nourish and support our body can be a rewarding and beneficial part of the emotional and spiritual stocktaking that we may naturally wish to do in this period of our lives.

MENOPAUSE AND HRT

Although I believe in the powerful effect that diet, supplements and lifestyle interventions can bring, I also believe in informed choice. Rather than a binary 'natural' versus 'medical' approach, I fully subscribe to an integrated approach in most areas, and this is especially true when it comes to HRT.

Having fallen out of favour, HRT has been having somewhat of a revival in the last few years thanks to improvements in the drugs available and better understanding of the potential risks and side effects. In some cases, the argument for HRT at certain, monitored windows of time are compelling. However, it is also known that simply taking HRT is not the full picture – the results are also linked to how well the body responds to, processes and clears that medicine once it has been absorbed, and this can be greatly influenced by our nutritional status. So whether you want to take HRT or not, a holistic, joined-up approach is key and all the recommendations in this chapter can support you – wherever you are in your journey.

Supplements

Multi-nutrient for your life stage – For all-round vitamin and mineral support. This should include zinc to balance testosterone, vitamin B6 for energy and hormone regulation, and vitamin D, which helps to regulate sex hormones.

Omega 3 – This contributes to wellbeing on many levels, including supporting mood, reducing inflammation, helping brain function and reducing menstrual cramping. Take 1g per day.

Soya isoflavones – Isoflavones can help to mitigate the symptoms associated with hormonal changes during menopause. 50–100mg once a day.

Ashwagandha – KSM ashwagandha has been shown to reduce stress, anxiety and insomnia, as well as weight management and healthy ageing.

I fully advocate herbal medicine at this stage in life and recommend looking for a combination of herbs that have been shown to support women during perimenopause and menopause, including dong quai, sage and hops. Speak to a herbal practitioner for advice specific relating to your symptoms and experience.

 Testing

If you suspect you are experiencing iron deficiency, you can get this tested at your GP surgery.

Hormone screening can also be helpful if you suspect you may be menopausal or may have a thyroid issue that is contributing to your symptoms. You are able to get a hormone screening (including your thyroid hormones) completed at your GP surgery. However, these may not be comprehensive enough for your symptoms and can be quite crude – ruling out borderline conditions or life stages, depending on the time of cycle completed, such as perimenopause. More comprehensive hormone screening is available through private laboratories under the guidance of the nutritional therapist or naturopath. They will also help you to interpret the results and create a supportive plan.

FERTILITY

Whether you are planning your first pregnancy or thinking about having another child, trying to conceive naturally or undergoing fertility treatment, the period of time before you conceive gives you a window of opportunity to evaluate your nutrition and general lifestyle.

Very often, fertility preparation is seen as the preserve of women. In fact, for over half the couples in the UK who experience subfertility (i.e. they are less than normally fertile), it is the result of problems on the male side.

If you and your partner know you want to conceive, you should both try to make some dietary changes three months ahead of that time. During these months, immature eggs, known as oocytes, mature in preparation for release during ovulation and sperm cells develop prior to ejaculation. Eating a nutritious diet during this time greatly influences the quality and efficiency of this process and gives you an even greater opportunity to create a healthy pregnancy.

Making dietary changes and improving nutrient stores may also help to correct factors that may be affecting your ability to conceive, such as a low sperm count in men or hormonal imbalances during the menstrual cycle in women.

Building a relationship with your baby can start before you conceive. Investing in and caring for your health during the preconception period will provide your baby with a nutrient-rich environment in which to thrive from day one of pregnancy. It is the window of opportunity for you to start building the nutrient reserves for *your* experience of a healthy pregnancy too, to minimise your experience of common pregnancy ailments and make pregnancy the enjoyable, blossoming journey that it can be.

Nutrition is the foundation for you and your baby

Studies have shown that couples who have made changes to their diet and lifestyle improved their chances of having a healthy pregnancy and baby, but research has shown that the benefits extend way beyond this. Indeed, how healthy your diet and lifestyle are during the preconception period is now understood to sow the seeds of health for your growing baby in infancy, such as reducing the risk of atopic conditions like asthma and eczema, and chronic health conditions in adulthood, such as diabetes.

Eating a healthy diet before you conceive can also influence milk production during breastfeeding and reduce the potential of postnatal depression. Studies have shown that couples who took nutritional supplements to support a healthy diet had quicker conception rates than those who did not. Below are the nutrients that have been shown to support fertility in both men and women, so look for them when choosing your fertility supplement:

B vitamins

The entire B vitamin family is important during conception and pregnancy. However, vitamin B6 has been shown to support cycle regularity and redress imbalances in hormonal conditions such as fibroids, endometriosis and PMS. Research has shown that giving B6 to women who have trouble conceiving increases fertility. Vitamin B12 has been shown to improve low sperm count.

Zinc

This is an important mineral for its contribution to normal fertility and reproduction, cell division and protection of cells from general wear and tear. Zinc also contributes to normal DNA synthesis – the genetic material that forms the basis of all of us. Zinc deficiency is common (especially in those women with a history of taking the contraceptive pill) and can affect sperm and egg production. Good sources of zinc include pulses such as chickpeas, pumpkin seeds, cashews and almonds, meat, dairy, eggs and wholegrains.

L-methionine

All amino acids perform a vital role in good health and egg production. However, L-methionine is an essential amino acid that plays a role in hormone stability and therefore supports a regular menstrual cycle. It also protects cellular DNA from damage in the months before you conceive. Good sources are chicken, fish, tofu and quinoa.

Beta-carotene

There has been concern about excess intake of vitamin A, a fat-soluble nutrient, in the form of retinol during pregnancy. The vegetable source of vitamin A, beta-carotene, is converted to vitamin A in the body as and when your body needs it, so there is no risk of an excess amount being produced. The corpus luteum, a hormonal structure that produces progesterone after a woman has ovulated, has the highest concentration of beta-carotene in the body. So beta-carotene can influence cycle regularity and the early stages of pregnancy. Good sources are carrots, sweet potatoes, tomatoes, spinach and broccoli.

Vitamin D

The latest research has demonstrated how important sufficient vitamin D is for a healthy conception and pregnancy, as well as to reduce the risk of gestational diabetes. Getting enough vitamin D can be hard through diet and sunshine alone (especially if you live at a more northerly latitude) and so supplements can be a good support. Good sources are dairy, eggs and oily fish.

Vitamin E

This is another antioxidant shown to benefit fertility in both men and women. Supplementing with vitamin E during IVF treatment has been found to improve fertilisation rates. Good sources are sunflower seeds, almonds and wheat bran.

Selenium

A healthy level of this trace mineral has been shown to improve low sperm count and healthy sperm formation. As an antioxidant, it also reduces the risk of miscarriage caused by chromosomal abnormalities. Good sources are Brazil nuts, wholegrain rice, shellfish and eggs.

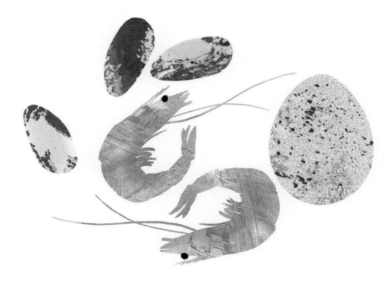

Folic acid

Along with other members of the B vitamin family, such as B12, folic acid is used to produce the important genetic material of the egg and the sperm in the three months prior to conception. Folic acid deficiency has been linked to a developmental abnormality known as a neural tube defect (such as spina bifida), which arises between the 24th and 28th day after conception. Supplementation in the three months before you conceive and during the first 12 weeks of pregnancy lowers this risk by 70 per cent, as well as reducing the risk of 'small for gestational age' babies and cleft lip and palate (De-Regil et al., 2010). The recommendation is for folate to be taken in the 12 weeks prior to conception because once you are pregnant, your baby's supply of folate is drawn from the reserves you have built up over the three months before you conceive. Good sources are broccoli, chickpeas and leafy green vegetables.

Vitamin C
This antioxidant had been shown to reduce excess histamine, which can inhibit the body's production of cervical mucus. This mucus supports the sperm in reaching the cervix. Vitamin C also acts as a protectant against sperm damage. Good sources are sweet potatoes, tomatoes, citrus fruits and broccoli.

Chromium and inositol
These lesser-known nutrients play a role in blood glucose management. Imbalances in blood glucose create a 'stress' response in the body, which can lower the chances of conception. Good sources are wholegrains such as rice and quinoa, and oranges.

Choline
This member of the B vitamin family supports normal liver function and how well your body breaks down fats. Liver health significantly affects hormone balance in both men and women. Choline also plays a central role in the unborn baby's brain development. Good sources are eggs, chicken and dairy foods.

Co-enzyme Q10
Recent research has shown that co-enzyme Q10 protects eggs and sperm from damage, as well as supporting healthy cell division in the first stages of pregnancy. Good sources are meats (especially poultry), eggs, oily fish and pulses like lentils.

Omega 3 fatty acids
These essential fats support hormone balance and the absorption of fat-soluble nutrients, such as vitamins E, D and K. They also form a

large part of the head of sperm and can therefore influence sperm quality and mobility. Good sources are oily fish, eggs and flaxseeds.

⌣ ☀ Diet and Lifestyle

Becoming as healthy as possible before you conceive is about nourishing your mind as well as your body.

Stress
Stress is not the preserve of the overworked, as often thought. Factors such as lack of sleep, dissatisfaction with where you are in your life and exercising too little or too much, are all potential stressors to the body. Whatever the reason for your stress, following the nutritional advice in this book can improve how well your body responds to it.

When you are stressed, your body adopts a fight, flight or freeze response. This triggers the release of the stress hormones cortisol and adrenaline, which affects digestion, blood pressure, circulation and brain function, and, over time, other areas of health, such as hormone balance and nutrient levels.

Creating opportunities to unwind – whether by doing yoga, massage, meditation or making small tweaks to your everyday routine, such as walking in your lunch hour or going to bed earlier – is an important part of encouraging relaxation and therefore combating stress. This is especially helpful during the fertility journey but also during pregnancy and parenthood.

Caffeine
Caffeine, especially in the form of coffee, has been shown to have a direct effect on fertility in some men and women. Although UK government guidelines suggest an intake of up to 200mg of caffeine a day (the equivalent of two cups of instant coffee) is

not harmful, a 2022 study indicated that drinking as little as one cup of coffee a day can decrease fertility and increase the risk of miscarriage by up to 50 per cent (Jafari et al., 2022). Caffeine has been found to adversely affect sperm count and motility and increase sperm abnormalities.

As well as coffee, caffeine is found in tea and fizzy drinks. There is also research into other ingredients found in these drinks, such as the stimulant theobromine, which is also present in decaffeinated versions. If you are trying to conceive, I recommend that you and your partner reduce your consumption of caffeinated and decaffeinated drinks, including coffee, colas, diet colas, chocolate and tea, with the exception of the odd cup of coffee or tea.

Alcohol

Alcohol can affect both male and female fertility. The *British Medical Journal* reported that women who had fewer than five units of alcohol a week were twice as likely to become pregnant in a six-month period than those women who drank more than this. Current recommendations by the Food Standards Agency (FSA) suggest limiting alcohol intake altogether during the preconception period and, if you do drink, have no more than one to two units once a week.

In men, alcohol can inhibit sperm count, motility and quality, and I recommend drinking fewer than six units per week. Additionally, alcohol can affect hormone balance, as well as reducing nutrient stores of key minerals for fertility, such as zinc (see page 185).

There are times when a having a lovely glass of wine can be part of a balanced lifestyle – when you are celebrating a special occasion, for example – but my advice is to treat alcohol mindfully. Respect the research highlighted above and, when you do drink alcohol, never do so on an empty stomach – this can adversely affect how well your body responds to and metabolises the alcohol.

Environmental factors

Environmental exposure to toxins from pesticides and plastics has been shown to impact on hormone balance and sperm production. The main culprit is a group of chemicals called xenoestrogens, which have a similar structure to the natural hormone oestrogen and contribute to hormonal imbalance. One of the best ways to eliminate an excess intake of these in the months before you conceive is to eat organic produce, particularly grains, fruit and vegetables you do not peel, such as berries and broccoli, as well as meat and dairy.

Toxic metals, such as mercury and lead, may also impact fertility in both men and women. These can be found in pesticides and oily fish, and there is a small amount in amalgam dental fillings. Additionally, exposure to other chemicals and toxic metals found in cigarettes have also been shown to impact on healthy development of the unborn baby. This is the ideal time to find the support you need to give up smoking for both you and your partner.

Medication can influence our nutrient levels too. For example, metformin, a drug given to people with type 2 diabetes, can reduce stores of vitamin B12; the contraceptive pill can reduce vitamin B6 and healthy bacteria in the gut; and statin medication for high cholesterol reduces co-enzyme Q10 stores.

For more information on these important environmental factors, I recommend you look at the website for Foresight Preconception (www.foresight-preconception.org.uk).

The importance of good liver health

The hormonal balance needed for fertility depends on good liver function. Aside from its daily task of detoxifying substances, such as caffeine and environmental toxins, the liver also chemically alters an excess of unused hormones. If this process does not happen effectively, hormonal imbalances can occur, affecting fertility and other health concerns, such as endometriosis, acne, premenstrual syndrome (PMS) and polycystic ovary syndrome (PCOS).

Supplements

A natural supplement – designed for preconception for you and your partner, which includes all of the nutrients recommended above.

Omega 3 fatty acids – 1g per day providing at least 400mg of DHA for both partners.

PREGNANCY AND EARLY MOTHERHOOD

Pregnancy

P regnancy is a wonderful opportunity to prioritise your complete wellbeing, to re-evaluate how you look after yourself in body and mind, and to start building a nurturing relationship with your baby. Research has shown that the quality of a mother's diet before she conceives and during pregnancy produces lifelong effects that can improve her baby's resistance to infection and degenerative disease later in life. Eating well in pregnancy is thought not only to benefit the baby but their subsequent children too. We would hope for pregnancy to be a joyful time, but it can also be a time of anxiety and uncertainty for many, particularly first-time mums, as we deal with often conflicting advice and sometimes the less pleasant side effects of growing new life, such as nausea, tiredness and discomfort. When much can feel out of our control, I think it can be comforting to know that by simply eating a healthy and nutritious diet you are supporting your baby's future health and that of their children too.

Key advice for pregnant women

Swap simple carbohydrates for complex carbohydrates
Stabilising your blood sugar is a key part of healthy eating during pregnancy. It will support your energy levels, reduce the incidence of symptoms such as morning sickness, reduce the risk of gestational diabetes and support your body's response to the hormonal changes that occur. For example, choose porridge instead of ready-made cereals; apples, pears and berries to deal with sweet cravings; and beans and wholegrains over white rice or pasta.

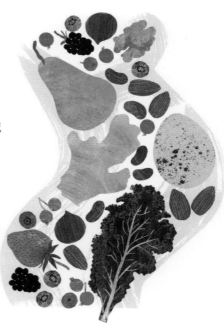

Eat a source of protein at each meal and snack
All protein is made up of amino acids, which are the basic building blocks of all human tissue. So, as you can imagine, protein is very important when building a new human being! Protein is needed for the growth of your unborn baby and the placenta, as well as to support the hormonal changes that occur during pregnancy. Amino acids also form the enzymes necessary for the digestive processes, which can affect how well you absorb other nutrients from your food. Protein continues to be of great importance after the birth because it is also needed for the production of breastmilk. An egg for breakfast, a handful of nuts for snacking on during the day and lean meat, fish and pulses for dinner will all contribute to this.

Minimise or preferably avoid eating processed foods and sugary or diet drinks
Some contain caffeine and many unwanted chemicals. Apart from anything else, they will do you no favours in delivering you the nutrients you need or regulating your blood sugar levels. See pages 62–3 for more on the latter.

Focus on iron-rich foods
As with all nutrients during pregnancy, you are sharing your iron stores with your baby. Iron is in high demand throughout pregnancy, and especially towards the end of the pregnancy and post birth. Building in iron-rich foods helps to prevent your increased blood volume from causing you to develop anaemia.

Keep hydrated
Most adults need 6–8 glasses of water (about 1.2–1.5 litres) a day and while you are pregnant or breastfeeding, you will likely find that you need more. Drinking enough is a challenge when you're either feeling or being sick. Try your best to maintain your fluids by regularly sipping water, herbal and ginger teas. A useful tip is to consume a variety of seasonal soups, as this will help your nutrient intake while increasing your fluids.

Eat foods rich in omega 3
The reality is that fats are the powerhouse for every cell in your body and those of your baby, too. This is especially so for brain development because over 60 per cent of the brain is made of fat. The unborn baby's brain goes through significant growth during the first and third trimester. A good supply of healthy fats is therefore crucial for optimum development, and also important to build stores for breastfeeding and your recovery after the birth. In fact, research has shown that improving your intake of the essential fats (omega 3 and omega 6) can reduce the risk of your baby having a premature birth or a low birth weight and of you getting postnatal depression (Middleton, 2018). If you do not have enough, the placenta draws

from the mother's DHA/EPA stores, concentrating stores in the body to that of twice the level of the mother's. Eating fats is also important to support your intake of fat-soluble nutrients, such as vitamins A, D, E and K, as well as the fat-soluble plant compounds such as carotenes that can support the immune system.

Manage your symptoms with calcium, magnesium and vitamin D
Calcium works with vitamin D and magnesium to prevent muscle cramps, which can affect women during pregnancy, and to provide energy. Pasteurised cheese, nuts, green vegetables and wheatgerm are good sources of calcium and magnesium, while vitamin D is produced in the skin from sunlight and small amounts are available from oily fish and eggs.

MORNING SICKNESS

Pregnancy nausea, also known as morning sickness, affects about half of all pregnant women and, far from being confined to the morning, can actually occur all day. The tips in this chapter will support morning sickness generally, but if you are finding it hard to manage proper meals, think 'little and often' and prioritise rest more than normal. Vitamin B6 will support hormonal balance while helping to regulate your blood glucose, so try to eat foods such as organic turkey, chicken and beef, avocado, sunflower seeds and sesame seeds. I recommend taking a pregnancy multi-nutrient if you are struggling to hold things down, but if you feel you need more, consult the advice of a nutritional therapist.

Ginger can be very useful to reduce the feeling of nausea. Grate fresh ginger into hot water and leave to infuse for three minutes before sipping. A teaspoon of apple cider vinegar in 250ml of hot water can also be very helpful. Ensure you use organic apple cider vinegar with the 'mother'.

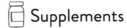 Supplements

A good-quality pregnancy multi-nutrient – containing 10mcg of vitamin D, 400mcg folic acid (in the form of natural folate), iodine and iron.

Omega 3 – 1g per day. Ratio of 1:2 EPA to DHA with at least 400mg of DHA. Concerns with oily fish consumption during pregnancy (due to the presence of toxic metals such as mercury and PCB pollutants) make supplementation an important choice for most.

Birth and beyond

I talk about pregnancy as the start of building your relationship with the miraculous human being you are growing. The fourth trimester, the first 12 weeks after your baby is born, is an extension of these foundations. A time to focus on and meet your needs through a nourishing diet, rest and permission to take life more gently.

If you are breastfeeding, a healthy diet is needed to support your supply of quality breastmilk, and of course it's important for you too. The right diet and adequate rest helps to restore hormonal balance after pregnancy, replenishes nutrient stores that have been diminished and supports your immune system and energy so that you can thrive and flourish too.

You have just been through a life-changing event and are probably feeling a confusing array of things – joy, discomfort and love, as well as being swollen, scared and in awe of your incredible body – probably all at once. With an overwhelming surge of hormones, the first 12 weeks can be particularly daunting.

After the birth

Your body will have been depleted by pregnancy and labour yet needs to be in peak physical condition for the challenge of nurturing an infant. You can support your body with a wide range of nutrients. Here are the headline things to bear in mind:

* **Antioxidants** will nourish stretched skin and help damaged tissues to recover from any tearing or from a caesarean.

* **Iron** can replenish stores after blood loss.

* **Calcium and magnesium** will replace that used up during muscle contractions.

* **B vitamins** can help you to stay calm and relaxed; they may be depleted from the high energy expenditure of birth and from any stress.

* **Zinc, vitamin D and essential fatty acids** are all protective against postnatal depression.

Food may be the last thing on your mind, but it has a beautiful way of grounding and healing you, providing nutrients to set you up for this next chapter in your life. Getting into a good routine is important but will be different for everyone and can take some trial and error. Here are a few tips to get you on the right track and make sure you are including all the key nutrients from the list above:

Keep it simple
It is at this stage you will reap the benefits of stocking up your postnatal storecupboard and utilising any pre-made frozen dishes that friends or family can provide. If you give birth during the wintery, damper months, avoid eating lots of cold foods and treat yourself to warming stews and soups. Slow-cooked foods can be very nourishing for the gut and immune system, as well as providing a little bit of

comfort. (I do recommend investing in a slow cooker if you don't have one already – see page 33 for more on the benefits of this style of cooking.) Eating in this way has also been shown to be supportive for postnatal mood too. When blood sugar levels are unstable and low, depression and anxiety can feel worse. Don't feel ashamed to ask for others' help in making nourishing meals in the early days. In many cultures, this is the standard practice with the mother focusing on rest and bonding with their new baby for the first weeks and months.

Prioritise iron- and zinc-rich foods

As birth can cause blood loss, it's important to replenish those stores, for energy, repair and immune health. Good sources of iron at this time include nettle tea, green leafy vegetables, oats, pulses, spinach, organic red meat and lentils. Remember to always pair plant iron with vitamin C-rich foods to aid absorption.

Zinc is needed for the immune system and healing after birth. It also supports the production and therefore the moderation of hormones, which will be very changeable over the next few weeks. It can also have an effect on symptoms of postnatal depression and has been shown to be especially effective in women who have been unresponsive to antidepressant medication. Build plenty of zinc-rich foods, such as nuts, lamb and wholegrains, into your diet.

Help your gut flourish

If you had medication during birth or a caesarean section, or lacked diversity in your diet while pregnant, your gut-friendly bugs may have taken a hit. Add probiotic foods such as sauerkraut, kefir and miso (a cup with warm water works well) to help repopulate or include a probiotic with lactobacillus strains (If breastfeeding, these will also help populate your baby's newly growing gut flora too.) Consider taking a probiotic supplement specific for pregnancy or breastfeeding, too.

Remember those all-important omega 3s

As I spoke about in the pregnancy section, during the third

trimester and while breastfeeding, your baby pulls on your stores of omega 3. Optimal levels are important for brain health, including memory and concentration, which may already be taking a hit if you are feeling sleep deprived! Rich sources are sardines, mackerel, anchovies, salmon, herring, trout.

Breastfeeding

Breastmilk contains essential fatty acids, so it is important to replenish these in your diet if you are breastfeeding your baby. They are needed for healthy hormone balance and to protect against fatigue, allergies and the memory loss and confusion that is often attributed to tiredness after birth. Breastmilk will provide your baby with friendly gut bacteria that will make vitamin K once they have fully populated their digestive system.

Supplements for breastfeeding mothers

A good-quality natural multi-nutrient – Some companies formulate their pregnancy supplement so that it contains all of the nutrients needed in breastfeeding too. Ensure it contains vitamin B12 and calcium to support your nervous system, as well as iron and zinc to promote psychological wellbeing during the ups and downs of new motherhood.

Fenugreek and stinging nettle have traditionally been used for centuries to optimise milk supply and quality for lactating women.

Omega 3 – Look for a supplement of 1g per day providing at least 400mg of DHA. This will be required to support the quality of your breastmilk and provide essential fatty acids for your baby's developing nervous system and brain.

POSTNATAL DEPRESSION

The causes of postnatal depression can range from sudden changes in hormones to a traumatic birth. It is more than 'the baby blues' – it is debilitating and all-consuming. It can leave you feeling lethargic and hopeless, and disinterested in the baby and in taking care of yourself. It can affect appetite and sleep patterns and cause you to cry a lot. It lasts for several weeks and can occur at any stage in the first year of motherhood. It is important to remember that you are not alone and that help is available, including nutritional changes that can contribute to your healing. Do ask for help – there will be people who want to listen and support you to find balance again so that you can enjoy your baby and motherhood.

There is a significant body of research underlining the influence that healthy DHA and EPA intake can have on the reduction of symptoms of depression, both on their own and in combination with antidepressant medication. Studies are not conclusive, but there is sufficient evidence to indicate that they may help. A study conducted by the National Institute for Health and Care Excellence found that a 1 per cent increase in blood levels of DHA related to a 59 per cent decrease in the risk of depressive symptoms postnatally. Studies also show that in countries where fish intake is low, postnatal depression is higher. As unborn babies accumulate an average of 67mg of DHA per day in the last trimester, this can sometimes be at the cost of the mother's fatty acid stores postnatally.

Taking omega 3 fish oil supplements from the twentieth week of pregnancy to three months after the birth has been shown to be beneficial in improving mood.

However, these benefits were not seen in those women consuming omega 3 from plants or seeds sources. Therefore, if you are vegetarian or vegan, I recommend you support your diet with omega 3 supplements made from algae.

If you are struggling, then it is unlikely that a supplement will solve everything, but this information can be helpful to know. Again, please do ask for help. Be gentle with yourself, with your body and with your internal thoughts. You have already done an incredible job.

Supplements

Good-quality multi-nutrient for new mothers – A full multivitamin and mineral supplement offers the ideal foundations needed throughout the first 12 weeks of motherhood. Look for 400ug of folic acid in the form of natural folate and 400iu/10ug of vitamin D for healthy bones and teeth, as well as zinc, vitamin B12, iron, vitamin C, calcium and beta-carotene.

A broad-spectrum probiotic – to help repopulate your gut with lactobacillus strains to support the amount and diversity of your gut bacteria. If breastfeeding, these will also help populate your baby's growing gut flora. Include foods such as sauerkraut, kefir and miso too.

Omega 3 – In a ratio of 2:1 DHA to EPA and providing at least 400mg of DHA (see page 57). During the third trimester and while breastfeeding, your baby pulls on your stores. Optimal levels are important for brain health.

References

Barker, M. et al. (2018) 'Intervention strategies to improve nutrition
    and health behaviours before conception', *The Lancet*, (391), 5 May

Blume, C. et al. (2019) 'Effects of light on human circadian rhythms, sleep
    and mood', *Somnologie* (23): 147–156

Bundy, R. et al. (2004), 'Artichoke Leaf Extract reduces symptoms of
    Irritable Bowel Syndrome and improves life in otherwise healthy
    volunteers suffering from concomitant dyspepsia', *Journal of
    Alternative and Complementary Medicine*, (10), Aug: 667–9

Chang, JP. et al. (2019) 'High-dose eicosapentaenoic acid (EPA) improves
    attention and vigilance in children and adolescents with attention
    deficit hyperactivity disorder (ADHD) and low endogenous EPA
    levels', *Translational Psychiatry*, (9), 20 Nov

De-Regil, LM. et al. (2015) 'Effects and safety of periconceptional oral
    folate supplementation for preventing birth defects', *Cochrane
    Database of Systematic Reviews*, (12), 14 Dec

Gershon, M. (2020) *The Second Brain*, Harper Perennial, New York

Gundogdu, A. et al. (2023), 'The role of the Mediterranean diet in
    modulating the gut microbiome', *Nutrition*, (114), Oct

Jafari, A. et al. (2022) 'Relationship between maternal caffeine and coffee
    intake and pregnancy loss', *Frontiers in Nutrition*, (9), 9 Aug

Markowska, A. (2022) 'Immunohistochemical Expression of Vitamin D
    Receptor in Uterine Fibroids', *Nutrients*, (14), 17 Aug

Marziali, M. (2012) 'Gluten-free diet: a new strategy for management of painful
    endometriosis related symptoms?', *Minerva Chir.* (67), Dec: 499–504.

Matsuzaki, H. (2013) 'Antidepressant-like effects of a water-soluble
    extract from the culture medium of Ganoderma lucidum mycelia in
    rats', *BMC Complement Altern Med.* (13), 26 Dec

Matten, G. et al. (2012) *The Health Delusion: How to Achieve Exceptional
    Health in the 21st Century*, Hay House, London

Mental Health Foundation, *Sleep Matters: The impact of sleep on health
    and wellbeing*, 2011

Middleton, P. et al. (2018), 'Omega-3 fatty acid addition during pregnancy',
    Cochrane Database of Systematic Reviews 2018, (11), 15 Nov

Neumark-Sztainer, D. (2011), *"I'm, Like, SO Fat!": Helping Your Teen Make
    Healthy Choices about Eating and Exercise in a Weight-Obsessed World*,
    The Guildford Press: UK

Parazzini, F. et al. (2017) 'Magnesium in the gynaecological practice: a literature review', Magnes Res. (30) 1 Feb: 1–7

Rusu, E. et al. (2019) 'Prebiotics and Probiotics in atopic dermatitis', *Experimental and Therapeutic Medicine*, (18), Aug: 926–931

Srivastava, SB. (2021), 'Vitamin D: Do We Need More Than Sunshine?', *American Journal of Lifestyle Medicine*, (15), Jul–Aug

Srour, B. et al. (2021) 'Ultra-processed foods and human health', *The Lancet*, (31), 3 Feb

Tsaban, G. (2021) 'The effect of green Mediterranean diet on cardiometabolic risk', *Heart*, (107), 11 Jun: 1054–1061.

Vinson, JA. et al. (1988) 'Comparative bioavailability to humans of ascorbic acid alone or in a citrus extract', *American Journal of Clinical Nutrition* (48), Sept: 601–4

Wahl, S. et al. (2019) 'The Inner clock: Blue Light sets the human rhythm' *Journal of Biophotonics*, (12), 2 Sept

Wild Nutrition + The Future Laboratory (2022) *The Future of Perimenopause: Reclaiming a pivotal life stage*

Winter, H. et al. (2023) 'Can Dietary Patterns Impact Fertility Outcomes? A Systematic Review and Meta-Analysis', *Nutrients*, (15), 31 May: 2589

Yalçın Bahat, P. (2022) 'Dietary supplements for treatment of endometriosis: A review', *Acta Biomed.* (93), 14 Mar

Further Reading

Burke, I. (2016) *The Nature of Beauty*, Ebury Press: UK

Dimbleby, H. et al. (2024) *Ravenous: How to get ourselves and our planet into shape*, Profile Books: UK

Kumar, S. (2015) *Soil, Soil Society: A New Trinity for Our Time*, Ivy Press: UK

Lond-Caulk, T. (2022) *Eat Well and Feel Great: The Teenager's Guide to Nutrition*, Green Tree: UK

Newby, K. (2022) *The Natural Menopause Method*, HarperCollins: UK

Northrup, C. (2020) *Women's Health, Women's Wisdom*, Piatkus: UK

Norton, H. (2015) *Your Pregnancy Nutrition Guide*, Vermillion: UK

Pollan, M. (2009), *In Defence of Food: An Eater's Manifesto*, Penguin: USA

Rushton, E. (2022) *Natural Wellness Every Day*, Vermillion: UK

Van Tulleken, C. (2024) *Ultra-Processed People*, Penguin: UK

Welch, C. (2011) *Balance Your Hormones, Balance Your Life*, Da Capo Press: USA

Index

acne 96
adaptogens 67, 68, 75
adenomyosis 160–5
adolescence (12–19 years) 57–68
ageing 76–82
ALA (alpha-linolenic acid) 57
alcohol 131, 153–4, 174, 190
aloe vera 127
amenorrhea 166–70
anaemia 120–1
antioxidants 197
anxiety 102–4
ashwagandha 68, 75, 118, 183

bee products 156
beta-carotene 186
bioavailability 23
bioflavonoids 157
blood sugars 62–3, 111
blue light 109
body health 121–46
bone health 128–39
boswellia 138
breakfast 65
breastfeeding 199
busy adults, health hacks for 71–2

caffeine 111, 131, 137, 168, 174, 189–90
calcium 60–1, 67, 86–7, 195, 197

carbohydrates 36–7, 53, 136–7, 193
carotenoids 66, 143
cat naps 111
cholesterol 139–45
choline 188
chondroitin 138
chromium 188
co-enzyme Q10 188
colds 146–51
cooking 41

depression 104–5
DHA (docosahexaenoic acid) 56, 57, 74
diet, foundations of a healthy 29–39
digestion 80–1, 122–3, 127
drinks 35, 131, 194
dysmenorrhea 166–70

eczema 96–7
elderberries 151
emotions, 'eating' your 32
endometriosis 160–5
energy 112–17
environmental toxins 181, 191
EPA (eicosapentaenoic acid) 56, 74, 130, 135, 156
evening primrose oil 100, 169

exercise 38–9, 116, 131, 144, 148

fatigue 105–6
fats 37, 53, 66, 113, 142, 163, 168, 172, 179
fenugreek 199
fertility 184–92
fibre 53, 143, 173, 178
5HTP 119
flavours, variety of 35
flu 146–51
folic acid 187–8
Food-Grown® philosophy 25–6
food preparation 39–42
fried foods 137
fruit 40, 134–5, 167
fun 149

garlic 143
general health 146–58
ginger 143
glucosamine 138
glutamine 127
gluten 162
gut bacteria 144, 147, 155–6, 162, 168, 173, 178, 198
gut health 80–2, 114–15, 122–8

hay fever 151–8
hormesis effect 26

hormone screening 183
HRT (hormone
  replacement
  therapy) 182
hydration 35, 84,
  136, 194

IBS (irritable bowel
  syndrome) 123
infancy (0–12 months)
  47–9
inflammation 78
inositol 175, 188
intestinal permeability
  123–4
intolerances, food 128
iron 58–60, 84–5,
  101, 164, 194, 197,
  198
iron deficiency
  anaemia 120–1

joint pain 132–9

L-methionine 186
L-theanine 120
lavender 120
leaky gut syndrome
  123–4
light 109–10
liver health 191

magnesium 113, 118, 138,
  164, 169, 195, 197
mealtimes 37–8
meat, red 137
medication 18–19, 89
meditation 110
Mediterranean diet
  142–3

memory 111–12
menopause 175–83
menorrhagia 166–70
menstrual imbalances
  166–70
middle years 69–79
mind, healthy 101–21
mindfulness 110
mindset, eating with a
  nourishing 31
minerals 14–15, 21–2,
  162
mood 104–5, 112–17
morning sickness 195
motherhood 196–202
MSM 138
mushrooms, medicinal
  68, 75, 118, 150

NAC (N-acetyl-L-
  cysteine) 151
nightshade vegetables
  137
nutrients: natural 24–5
  nutrient-depletant
  foods 15–16
  synthetic 21–2
  why we aren't getting
  the right nutrients
  14–19

oestrogens,
  environmental 160,
  181
omega 3 fatty acids
  56–7, 66, 67, 74,
  85, 100, 118
for body health
  129, 135, 138, 139,
  143, 145

for general health
  149, 156
for women's health
  164, 168, 170, 182,
  188–9, 192, 194–5,
  196, 198–9, 202
organ meats 137
osteopenia and
  osteoporosis 128–32

PCOS (polycystic
  ovary syndrome)
  170–5
pectin 143
perimenopause 175–83
phytochemicals 131
phytoestrogens 163,
  168, 173, 178
picky eaters 55
plant sterols 141, 142
polyphenols 66
postnatal depression
  200–1
prebiotics 125–6
pregnancy 192–6
premenstrual
  syndrome (PMS)
  166–70
premenstrual tension
  (PMT) 166–70
preschool children
  49–51
probiotics 100, 119,
  124–5, 145, 147,
  155, 198, 201
processed foods 194
protein 36, 65, 83,
  113–14, 130, 174,
  178, 193
psoriasis 97–8

quercetin 157

rainbow diet 33–4, 66, 131, 148–9, 154, 161–2
reishi 68, 75, 118
rest 110
ripple effect 42

Safr'Inside™ saffron extract 119
St John's Wort 119
schoolchildren (5–12 years) 51–7
seasonal diet 33
selenium 187
skin health 95–101
sleep 39, 66, 106–17, 147–8, 180–1
slippery elm 127
smoking 131
soya isoflavones 183
spices 136, 154
spirituality 42–3
starflower oil 169
statins 145
stillness, practising daily 180
stinging nettles 199
stress 102–4, 134, 163–4, 168–9, 173, 180, 189
sugar 136–7, 142, 147, 174, 194
supplements 20–9
  added ingredients 29
  for bones and joint health 132, 138–9
  for breastfeeding 199
  for cholesterol 145
  for cold and flu 149–50
  for early adulthood to middle years 72
  for endometriosis and adenomyosis 164–5
  for fertility 192
  for gut health 127
  for hayfever 157–8
  for a healthy mind 117–20
  how to choose 27
  for infants (0–12 months) 49
  for menstrual disorders 169–70
  for middle years to wiser years 84–9
  natural vs synthetic 21
  for new mothers 201–2
  for PCOS 174–5
  for perimenopause and menopause 182–3
  for pregnancy 196
  RDA 27–8
  for schoolchildren (5–12 years) 56–7
  for skin health 100
  for teenagers 67
  for toddlers and preschoolers 50
  why we take 20

thyroid 101
tiredness 105–6
toddlers 49–51
toxins 181, 191
Tulsi 68

turmeric 138–9, 143, 151, 165

valerian root 119
vegans and vegetarians 36
vegetables 40, 134, 137, 163, 167, 178
vitamins 12–13, 21–2
  vitamin A 54–5
  B vitamins 88–9, 112–13, 117, 157, 185, 197
  vitamin B complex 175
  vitamin B3 145–6
  vitamin B6 157, 164, 170
  vitamin C 53–4, 113, 131, 143, 150, 157, 188
  vitamin D 56, 72–4, 85–6, 120, 129, 132, 139, 149, 172, 175, 186, 195, 197
  vitamin E 143, 186

weight 134, 181
Western diets 16–17
wiser years, middle years to 76–9
women's health 159–83

young adulthood 69–75

zinc 61–2, 100, 150, 156, 185, 197, 198

Acknowledgements

As in nature, a symbiosis of energy and effort created the writing on these pages. I owe great gratitude to Elen Jones for asking me to write this book; to Katherine Pitt, Tina Persaud, Liz Marvin and the entire team at Laurence King for their knowledge and encouragement; and to the incredible team at Wild Nutrition for their patience and support while I took myself away to write.

Thanks to you, the reader, for choosing this book. I hope that the information in these pages supports you in your understanding of natural nutrition and your body's needs, and encourages you to adopt simple and sustainable changes for a healthier life.

Finally, I am forever deeply grateful for, and inspired by, my very precious family of quite brilliant young men: Alfie, Ned and Oscar, and my treasured husband, Charlie. Your love and championing of my quests is the greatest gift of nourishment, and I feel the luckiest woman to receive it.

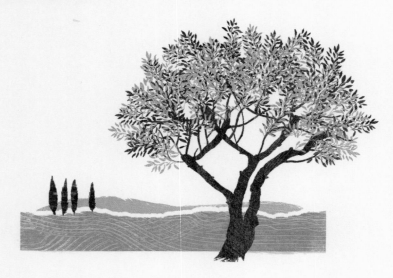